Publisher CompletelyKeto Corp.

This publication is designed to provide authoritative information in regard to the subject matter covered. Many of the product designations are clarified by trademarks. While every precaution has been taken in the preparation of this book, the author assumes no responsibility for errors or omissions, or damages resulting from the use of information contained herein. For additional information, please contact our support team:

https://CompletelyKeto.com/support

202102101PRFLPP

Table of Contents

$1,000 Bonus: Lifetime Support!

Join the Speed Keto™ Rapid Fat Loss Community here:

facebook.com/groups/speedketorfl

You will be asked for a code to join the group:

The code is RFLWORKS

You'll love the support in the group.

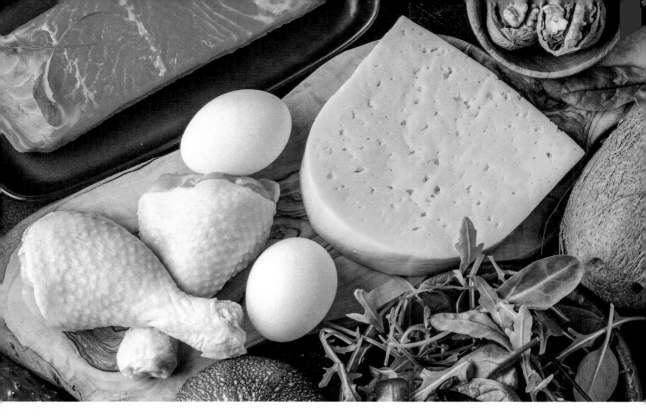

Disclaimer

Welcome and we're excited to have you with us on this journey. All of the information provided in the book and on the Websites located at completelyketo.com, completelyketo.shop, or speedketo.com or speedketo.shop is intended solely for general information and should NOT be relied upon for any particular diagnosis, treatment, or care. This book is not a substitute for medical advice. The book and websites are only for general informational purposes.

The information contained in this book is not a substitute for medical advice or treatment, and again the author strongly encourages patients and their families to consult with qualified medical professionals for treatment and related advice on individual cases.

Decisions relating to the prevention, detection, and treatment of all health issues should be made only after discussing the risks and benefits with your health care provider, considering your personal medical history, your current situation and your future health risks and concerns. If you are pregnant, nursing, diabetic, on medication, have a medical condition or are beginning a health or weight control program, consult your physician before using products or services discussed in this book and before making any other dietary changes. This diet is not recommended or supported for those under the age of eighteen. By using this book, you represent that you are at least eighteen (18) years old and a United States resident.

The authors cannot guarantee that the information in this book is safe and proper for every reader. For this reason, this book is offered without warranties or guarantees of any kind, expressed or implied, and the authors disclaim any liability, loss or damage caused by the contents, either directly or consequentially. The U.S. Food and Drug Administration or any other government regulatory body has not evaluated statements made in this book. Products, services, and methods discussed in this book are not intended to diagnose, treat, cure or prevent any disease.

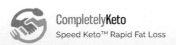

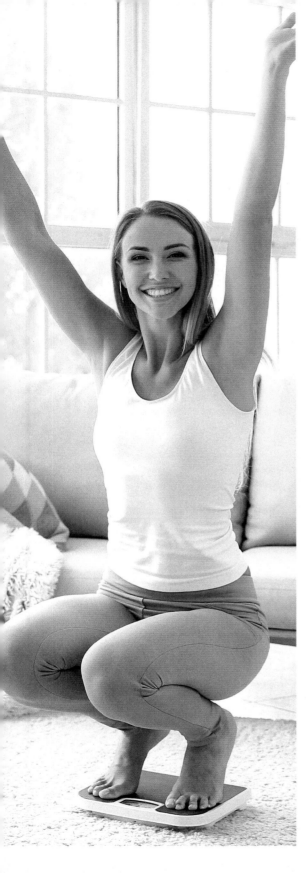

Introduction

This program is different than any other weight loss program. You will be stepping out of your comfort zone. The best thing about that is, when you switch up your methods, the body is kept guessing. Your system doesn't know what to expect, so it works harder and intensifies your results. This program is unlike any of the others, and that's a good thing!

We tracked over 100 users who followed the 28 day Rapid Fat Loss program. They reported their starting body weight and measurements and then reported the changes at the conclusion of the program. The average results were a staggering 22 pounds in 28 days. I hope one day a university will do a study of the results.

Each variation in every one of my weight loss programs is carefully planned to confuse the body's metabolic response. These changes not only promote fat burning, but they also cleanse the body of toxins and impurities that zap energy/fat burning potential. The best part is the elimination of inflammatory foods from your diet. The results are often dramatic in nature.

This program includes only sirtuin foods. Let's get into what those are. These are foods that activate specific genes in our body to burn fat more quickly. These sirtuin genes also preserve muscle. When activated, these specific genes mimic calorie restriction even when eating at maintenance calories. Then, we kick that fat burning up a notch with 3 unfasting days with lower calories, but plenty of high-quality nutrition.

Sirtuins are metabolic regulators. That's how they got the name, "skinny genes". Ramping these sirtuin genes up results in longevity, cellular health and reduced inflammation. These results go beyond vitamins and minerals. We are using actual food chemicals to regulate the bodies health by activating specific genes.

Our cells benefit from low grade beneficial stress on the body like fasting, sauna and exercise. Activating sirtuin genes mimics this low-grade beneficial stress. This activates a recycling of our cells. The buildup of toxins and fat will turn over and be released from the body much like they do when exercising and fasting.

CompletelyKeto
Speed Keto™ Rapid Fat Loss

This process pushes the body to quickly generate new cells. Your metabolism is super charged and is a more efficient fat burner. The body becomes a low insulin, low inflammation environment which allows more fat burning to take place.

Most of the medications used to treat diseases are derived from plants. One of the creators, a long time expert on natural healing, set out to pinpoint the exact foods that have beneficial properties. The idea is nutrition as a medicine, for not only curative means but preventative as well. They discovered that there were certain foods that activate sirtuin genes.

You'll be meeting these high nutrition fat-burning foods shortly.

> *We pride ourselves on our support.* You can get all of your questions answered by joining our fabulous Facebook group here: www.facebook.com/groups/speedketorfl or search on Facebook for Speed Keto™ RFL program. We offer unlimited support so for maximum success please join our group.

Water

Clean, filtered, purified water is essential to being successful in cleansing the body of toxins. You'll have your first 20 oz of water first thing in the morning. Have a bottle on the bedside table waiting for you. Drink those 20 oz right when you wake up, before you even get out of bed. Drinking this amount, at this time of day will flush out all the toxins that have been accumulated in the body over night while your system has been working. During sleep the body uses that time of rest to purge those systems working so hard during the day. This purge happens in the gut, the lymphatic system and even the skin.

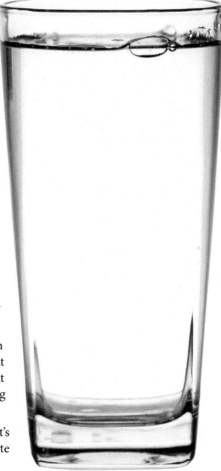

Only filtered or bottled water is allowed in this program. No alkaline water, fruit water, or carbonated water whatsoever. Refrigerator filters, Brita filters, etc., are allowed. Hint water is permitted.

You will drink, in total 100 oz, daily, of purified water. We are putting emphasis on purified water to eliminate impurities and contaminates. Those contaminates cause inflammation in the body. In this program we are cleansing and flushing out those impurities. Reducing contaminates and inflammation in the body is very important to your success. When you eliminate toxins and inflammation your body fat reduces. A clean system cycles fat out of the body instead of holding onto it.

While exercising you'll drink 10 oz every 15 minutes. When you exercise, your body sweats and purges impurities. That sweat is not only water, it is built up toxins and actual fat leaving the body. By continuing to drink water, you're helping your system eliminate those toxins faster.

After your daily High Intensity Interval Training (relax it's simple) exercise session is when you'll have your electrolyte drink. 1 scoop in 16 oz water per day.

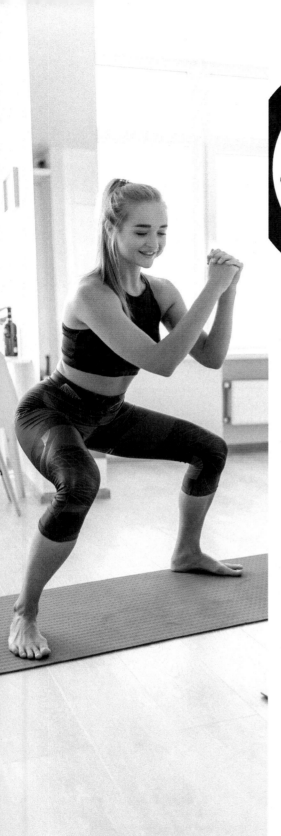

Unless you are exercising more than once a day, only drink one electrolyte scoop. You can also increase electrolytes, up to 3 times a day, if you are experiencing electrolyte imbalance symptoms. Overdoing the electrolyte drinks will cause your body to hold onto water weight so only increase if you need to.

Daily exercise

30 minutes of walking daily would be an added bonus but mainly we will be focusing on HIIT. High intensity interval training, the type of HIIT we will be doing is called Tabata. You can download a Tabata timer on your phone to help with your exercises. You will exercise as hard as you can for 20 seconds followed by 10 seconds of rest. Studies show this type of exercise packs a huge punch. In 4 minutes of HIIT you will have done the work of an hour of steady exercise.

Exercise as vigorously as you can for 20 seconds then stop 10 for seconds. These 20 seconds will be explosive in intensity. At the end of 4 minutes exercise will equal 1 hour of exercise. This will shed maximum weight. These exercises can be adjusted to your abilities. There are countless resources online for recommended HIIT workouts. They range from walking, running, body weight movements to gym equipment. The exercises you choose are up to you.

Twice a week we will be using 1-2 lb weights to accelerate fat burning. There are no excuses! If a part of your body is injured simply use the other part of your body. The purpose of this short yet explosive exercise is to get the lymphatic system moving and get the toxins out of your body.

Many people use my Just4Minutes program at just4minutes.com as a simple Tabata program.

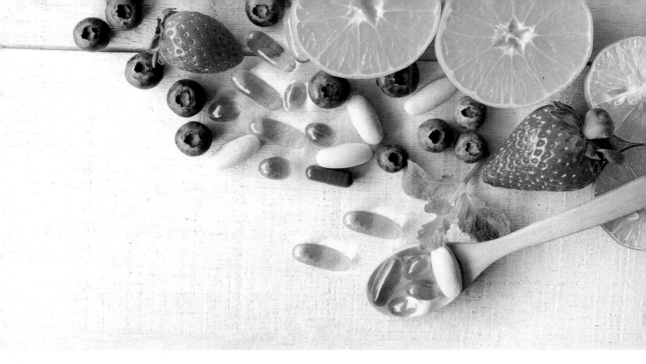

Supplements

Supplements are very important in this program. You'll be taking your supplements every day. All of the supplements are very important. You'll find links (and discounts) in the Facebook group.

Probiotics

Your probiotic is important to be taken on an empty stomach each morning. We need those good bacteria working for us in the gut all day long while we eat, move and go about the day. Gut health is imperative to overall body health. Taking your probiotic on an empty stomach, after your morning water allows a clean straight path directly to the gut. This way, when you eat your first meal, those good bacteria are waiting to work for you, helping the body use the nutrition it receives in the most efficient way.

Triphala

Triphala, as a powder or pill. It's all natural and detox safe. This supplement has been used for thousands of years. Take this supplement before bed to activate an inner cleanse while you sleep. You'll take 2 capsules or ¼ tsp in warm water before bed. Triphala is part of a health system called Ayurveda. In Ayurveda there are 3 body types and personality types.

- Doshas are the ayurvedic body types. (Vata, Pitta, Kapha)
- Vata embodies air and ether, this body type is often thin.
- Pitta embodies the transformative nature of fire and may be upset easily.
- Kapha reflects the binding nature of water energy and people with this body type are often overweight.

These supplements we recommend help to balance kapha.

There are 2 formulas for reducing kapha. You will only use one or other, not both. If you need to lose 50-100 pounds, kapha is the supplement you should use. If you need to lose more than 100 Pounds, Punarnava powder is best with warm water in the morning. These help to remove fat from the body. See the Facebook group for links.

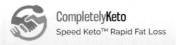

Digestive enzymes

Most people don't digest food properly. With aging, digestion slows considerably. Take digestive enzymes, 2 with every meal (multi spectrum enzyme). Enzymes help break down food and get more nutrients from the food you eat. The goal with everything we eat in this program is to absorb nutrients.

Activated charcoal

When there is a change in diet, the body does notice, and it may respond unfavorably for a short period of time but not to worry, your body will adjust! Have some activated charcoal on hand if your stomach becomes upset. It will calm your stomach rapidly. 2 charcoal pills will do the trick.

Sirt drinks

The internal/external metabolic boost drink is something you will have only on unfasting days, multiple times a day. The metabolic boost drink in our program is different from the one you will find in the traditional sirt food diet, because we have eliminated all of the sugar, leaving only the most important and beneficial nutrients. This drink can be juiced or simply made into a smoothie in a blender. If you have an allergy to any of the ingredients feel free to leave it out. You will have the anti-inflammatory drink every day.

(Green Drink) Internal/External Metabolic Boost Drink

- 1 large cucumber
- 1 cup alfalfa sprouts
- ½ bunch parsley
- 3-4 snips fresh mint
- ½ cup lemon or lime juice
- Drop of stevia (only if needed)

Anti-Inflammatory Drink

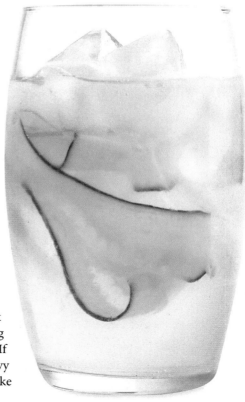

- 3 tbsp organic lemon juice
- 2 tsp organic turmeric powder
- 4 tsp ginger powder
- Dash black & cayenne pepper
- Up to 4 drops pure stevia
- Mixed into 4 oz water

Morning Coffee or Green Tea

In your morning coffee or tea add 1 scoop (1 tsp) of MCT oil or powder. This helps to accelerate your metabolism. These do not count toward your daily water goal. We are using foods that are nutritionally beneficial to us. If you absolutely must, you can use a drop of heavy whipping cream and or a drop of stevia. Make sure it's pure stevia.

Green Tea; Black Tea

Green tea is excellent for stimulating the metabolism. There are many proven benefits of green tea or matcha. Matcha is the same plant as green tea, only it is produced in a different way. We recommend matcha because it is far more nutrient dense than regular green tea. Farmers boost chlorophyl, antioxidant and amino acid production in the plant by blocking it from sunlight for 30 days prior to harvest. This is a beneficial stress to the plant which creates a healthier and stronger super food. Matcha helps to protect the liver, promotes heart health and increases fat loss by increasing metabolism.

Cocoa/Cacao

Cacao is known to lower blood pressure, reduce the risk of diabetes and promotes healthy digestion. It also reduces inflammation. In this program we have 1 tsp in hot water only on unfast days, 30 minutes before dinner. It fills you up so you aren't as hungry.

Wine

Red wine has sirtuins and resveratrol. We are only drinking dry red wine, Pinot Noir, Malbec or Cabernet, 5-6 oz. These are the ONLY types of wine allowed on this program. Wine is allowed only on eating days, not on unfasting days. You'll be able to enjoy wine 2 nights a week. We recommend Dry Farms or Fit Vines brands.

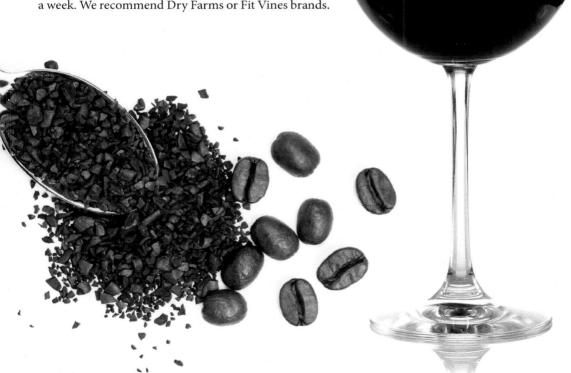

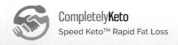

Completely**Keto**
Speed Keto™ Rapid Fat Loss

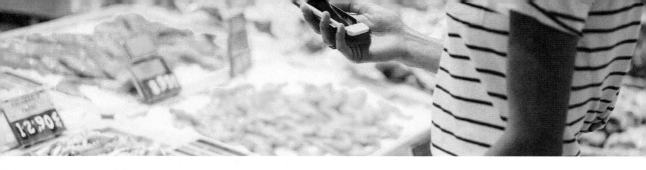

Nutrition

We will only be eating fresh whole foods. No processed keto foods. The exceptions are broths and Crepini egg thins. In order to cleanse and replenish our system we are avoiding all artificial food additives. The goal here is balanced meals made up of 3.5-4 oz of protein, 2-4 cups of vegetables.

Approved foods list

Protein ─────────────

- Beef
- Chicken
- Turkey
- Lamb
- White fish
- Salmon
- Tuna in water
- Eggs (up to 3 for lunch or dinner)
- Lobster
- Crab
- Shrimp
- Veal

Vegetables ─────────────

- Spinach
- Chard/swiss chard
- Chicory
- Field greens
- Arugula
- Kale
- Cabbage
- Broccoli
- Cauliflower
- Brussels sprouts
- Fennel
- French beans (string beans)
- Red/Green/Yellow peppers
- Zucchini
- Red radishes
- Cucumber
- Asparagus
- Mushrooms
- Red onions
- Celery
- Cherry tomatoes (after round one)

Additions ─────────────

- Wheat free tamari
- Primal Kitchen mayonnaise
- Primal Kitchen ketchup
- Mustard
- All spices and herbs, without sugar or oil
- Crepini Egg Thins
- Chicken/Beef/Bone broth
- Lilly's dark chocolate 85% or over
- Cocoa powder
- Green tea
- Coffee
- Pinot noir
- Malbec
- Cabernet

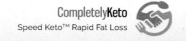

CompletelyKeto
Speed Keto™ Rapid Fat Loss

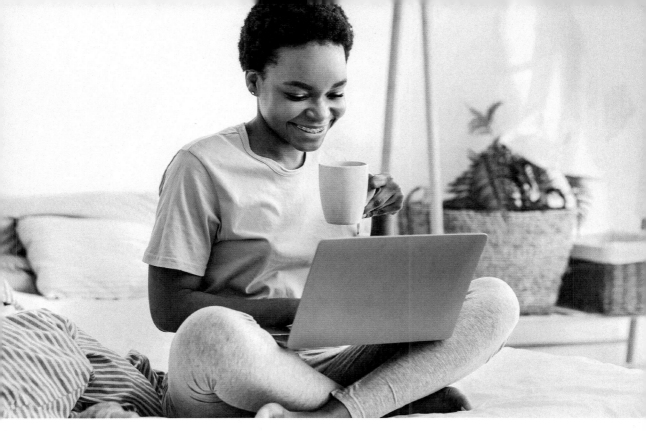

Unfasting days

We do intermittent fasting on this program, but it isn't a traditional fast so we call these days unfasting days. We are confusing metabolism with our unfasting. Unfasting days are Monday, Wednesday, Friday. No fast on weekends. Be sure to drink your 100 oz of water.

Here's your unfasting schedule.

- Wake up and drink 20 oz water.

- Exercise! 4 minutes of Tabata or go for a walk.

- Drink your electrolytes.

- Enjoy your morning coffee or matcha with 1 tsp MCT oil or 1 scoop MCT powder. Only use a drop of stevia or 1 tsp heavy whipping cream if necessary.

- Drink your AID – Anti-inflammatory drink.

- Take your supplements (Probiotic, kapha or Punarnava)

- Around lunch time drink your internal/external metabolic boost (green drink). You can have up to 3 of these on unfasting days.

- Drink beef, chicken or bone broth. Have as much as you like.

- 30 minutes before dinner drink your cocoa/cacao drink. (1 tsp in a cup of hot water)

- Take your digestive enzymes, then enjoy a delicious dinner!

- For dessert, eat a short row of approved chocolate. For Lilly's bars this will be 5 squares. For any other bar it will be 13.33g of chocolate.

- Take your Triphala before bed. 2 capsules or ¼ tsp of the powder in warm water.

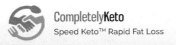

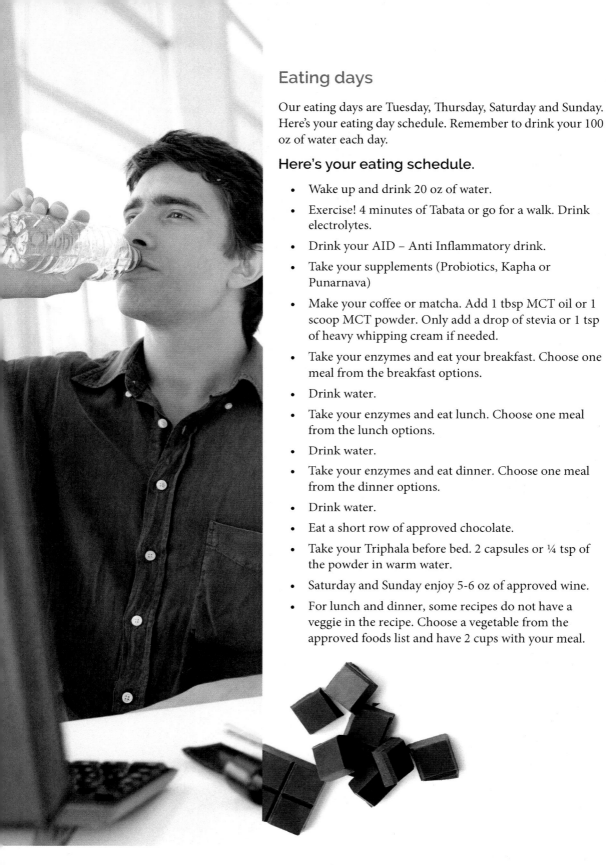

Eating days

Our eating days are Tuesday, Thursday, Saturday and Sunday. Here's your eating day schedule. Remember to drink your 100 oz of water each day.

Here's your eating schedule.

- Wake up and drink 20 oz of water.
- Exercise! 4 minutes of Tabata or go for a walk. Drink electrolytes.
- Drink your AID – Anti Inflammatory drink.
- Take your supplements (Probiotics, Kapha or Punarnava)
- Make your coffee or matcha. Add 1 tbsp MCT oil or 1 scoop MCT powder. Only add a drop of stevia or 1 tsp of heavy whipping cream if needed.
- Take your enzymes and eat your breakfast. Choose one meal from the breakfast options.
- Drink water.
- Take your enzymes and eat lunch. Choose one meal from the lunch options.
- Drink water.
- Take your enzymes and eat dinner. Choose one meal from the dinner options.
- Drink water.
- Eat a short row of approved chocolate.
- Take your Triphala before bed. 2 capsules or ¼ tsp of the powder in warm water.
- Saturday and Sunday enjoy 5-6 oz of approved wine.
- For lunch and dinner, some recipes do not have a veggie in the recipe. Choose a vegetable from the approved foods list and have 2 cups with your meal.

CompletelyKeto
Speed Keto™ Rapid Fat Loss

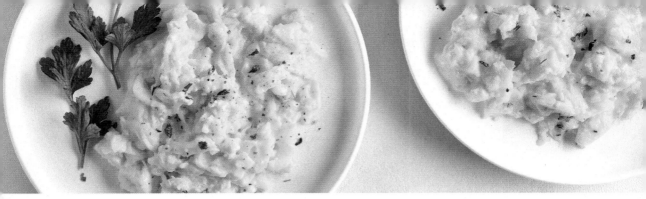

Week 1 ─────────────

Sunday

- Morning: 20 oz water, anti-inflammatory drink, supplements, coffee or tea with MCT
- Take enzymes before each meal and drink 100 oz of water today.
- Breakfast: Completely Keto Strawberry Shake
- Lunch: Tuna on a Log
- Dinner: Baked Mahi Mahi with Balsamic Glaze
- After dinner: One row of approved dark chocolate and 5-6 oz red wine
- Before bed: Triphala

Monday (Unfasting Day)

- Morning: 20 oz water, anti-inflammatory drink, supplements, coffee or tea with MCT.
- Take enzymes before dinner and drink 100 oz water today
- Lunch: Have your metabolic boost Green drink (you can have up to 3 of these today)
- Beef, chicken, bone broth (as much as you'd like)
- 30 minutes before dinner have cacao drink
- Dinner: Beef Skewers
- After dinner: One row of approved dark chocolate
- Before bed: Triphala

Tuesday

- Morning: 20 oz water, anti-inflammatory drink, supplements, coffee or tea with MCT
- Take enzymes before each meal and drink 100 oz of water today.
- Breakfast: 2 Scrambled Eggs
- Lunch: Chicken and Vegetable Kebabs
- Dinner: Spicy Chicken Wings
- After dinner: One row of approved dark chocolate
- Before bed: Triphala

Wednesday (Unfasting Day)

- Morning: 20 oz water, anti-inflammatory drink, supplements, coffee or tea with MCT.
- Take enzymes before dinner and drink 100 oz water today
- Lunch: Have your metabolic boost Green drink (you can have up to 3 of these today)
- Beef, chicken, bone broth (as much as you'd like)
- 30 minutes before dinner have cacao drink
- Dinner: Miami Short Ribs
- After dinner: One row of approved dark chocolate
- Before bed: Triphala

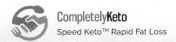

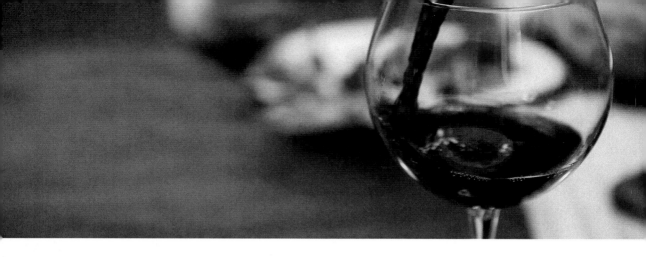

Thursday

- Morning: 20 oz water, anti-inflammatory drink, supplements, coffee or tea with MCT
- Take enzymes before each meal and drink 100 oz of water today.
- Breakfast: Spinach Omelet
- Lunch: Greek Salad
- Dinner: Crockpot Pulled Chicken
- After dinner: One row of approved dark chocolate
- Before bed: Triphala

Friday (Unfasting Day)

- Morning: 20 oz water, anti-inflammatory drink, supplements, coffee or tea with MCT.
- Take enzymes before dinner and drink 100 oz water today
- Lunch: Have your metabolic boost Green drink (you can have up to 3 of these today)
- Beef, chicken, bone broth (as much as you'd like)
- 30 minutes before dinner have cacao drink
- Dinner: Braised Lamb
- After dinner: One row of approved dark chocolate
- Before bed: Triphala

Saturday

- Morning: 20 oz water, anti-inflammatory drink, supplements, coffee or tea with MCT
- Take enzymes before each meal and drink 100 oz of water today.
- Breakfast: Tuna Stuffed Bell Pepper
- Lunch: Cauliflower, Broccoli, Bacon Salad
- Dinner: Simple Beef and Vegetable Soup
- After dinner: One row of approved dark chocolate and 5-6 oz red wine
- Before bed: Triphala

Week 2

Sunday

- Morning: 20 oz water, anti-inflammatory drink, supplements, coffee or tea with MCT
- Take enzymes before each meal and drink 100 oz of water today.
- Breakfast: Egg Salad on Bed of Spinach
- Lunch: Cucumber and Tuna Roll-ups
- Dinner: Lemon Garlic Chicken Breasts
- After dinner: One row of approved dark chocolate and 5-6 oz red wine
- Before bed: Triphala

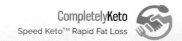

CompletelyKeto
Speed Keto™ Rapid Fat Loss

Monday (Unfasting Day)

- Morning: 20 oz water, anti-inflammatory drink, supplements, coffee or tea with MCT.
- Take enzymes before dinner and drink 100 oz water today
- Lunch: Have your metabolic boost Green drink (you can have up to 3 of these today)
- Beef, chicken, bone broth (as much as you'd like)
- 30 minutes before dinner have cacao drink
- Dinner: <u>Red Curry Zoodle Soup</u>
- After dinner: One row of approved chocolate
- Before bed: Triphala

Wednesday (Unfasting Day)

- Morning: 20 oz water, anti-inflammatory drink, supplements, coffee or tea with MCT.
- Take enzymes before dinner and drink 100 oz water today
- Lunch: Have your metabolic boost Green drink (you can have up to 3 of these today)
- Beef, chicken, bone broth (as much as you'd like)
- 30 minutes before dinner have cacao drink
- Dinner: <u>Beef and Cauliflower Burgers</u>
- After dinner: One row of approved dark chocolate
- Before bed: Triphala

Tuesday

- Morning: 20 oz water, anti-inflammatory drink, supplements, coffee or tea with MCT
- Take enzymes before each meal and drink 100 oz of water today.
- Breakfast: <u>Turkey and Cucumber Roll-ups</u>
- Lunch: <u>Beef Zomein</u>
- Dinner: <u>Kung Pao Chicken</u>
- After dinner: One row of approved dark chocolate
- Before bed: Triphala

Thursday

- Morning: 20 oz water, anti-inflammatory drink, supplements, coffee or tea with MCT
- Take enzymes before each meal and drink 100 oz of water today.
- Breakfast: <u>Smoked Salmon on Bed of Arugula</u>
- Lunch: <u>Chicken Kale Spinach Salad</u>
- Dinner: <u>Salmon Skewers</u>
- After dinner: One row of approved dark chocolate
- Before bed: Triphala

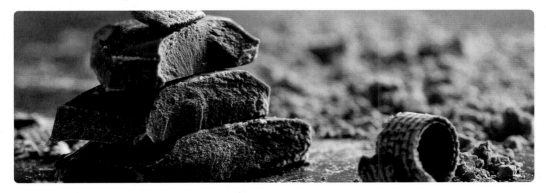

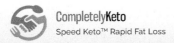

CompletelyKeto
Speed Keto™ Rapid Fat Loss

Friday (Unfasting Day)

- Morning: 20 oz water, anti-inflammatory drink, supplements, coffee or tea with MCT.
- Take enzymes before dinner and drink 100 oz water today
- Lunch: Have your metabolic boost Green drink (you can have up to 3 of these today)
- Beef, chicken, bone broth (as much as you'd like)
- 30 minutes before dinner have cacao drink
- Dinner: Pepper Steak
- After dinner: One row of approved dark chocolate
- Before bed: Triphala

Saturday

- Morning: 20 oz water, anti-inflammatory drink, supplements, coffee or tea with MCT
- Take enzymes before each meal and drink 100 oz of water today.
- Breakfast: Cabbage Hash Browns
- Lunch: Turkey Zucchini Burgers
- Dinner: Hunter's Stew
- After dinner: One row of approved dark chocolate and 5-6 oz red wine
- Before bed: Triphala

Week 3

Sunday

- Morning: 20 oz water, anti-inflammatory drink, supplements, coffee or tea with MCT
- Take enzymes before each meal and drink 100 oz of water today.
- Breakfast: Turkey Bacon and Zucchini
- Lunch: Beef Satay
- Dinner: Harlan Kilstein's Meatloaf
- After dinner: One row of approved dark chocolate and 5-6 oz red wine
- Before bed: Triphala

Monday (Unfasting Day)

- Morning: 20 oz water, anti-inflammatory drink, supplements, coffee or tea with MCT.
- Take enzymes before dinner and drink 100 oz water today
- Lunch: Have your metabolic boost Green drink (you can have up to 3 of these today)
- Beef, chicken, bone broth (as much as you'd like)
- 30 minutes before dinner have cacao drink
- Dinner: Sesame Crusted Salmon
- After dinner: One row of approved dark chocolate
- Before bed: Triphala

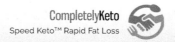

CompletelyKeto
Speed Keto™ Rapid Fat Loss

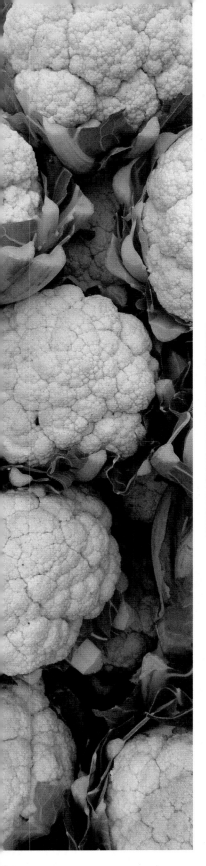

Tuesday

- Morning: 20 oz water, anti-inflammatory drink, supplements, coffee or tea with MCT
- Take enzymes before each meal and drink 100 oz of water today.
- Breakfast: <u>Bacon and Eggs</u>
- Lunch: <u>Chicken and Rice Soup</u>
- Dinner: <u>Grilled Skirt Steak</u> for 2
- After dinner: One row of approved dark chocolate
- Before bed: Triphala

Wednesday (Unfasting Day)

- Morning: 20 oz water, anti-inflammatory drink, supplements, coffee or tea with MCT.
- Take enzymes before dinner and drink 100 oz water today
- Lunch: Have your metabolic boost Green drink (you can have up to 3 of these today)
- Beef, chicken, bone broth (as much as you'd like)
- 30 minutes before dinner have cacao drink
- Dinner: <u>Club For One</u>
- After dinner: One row of approved dark chocolate
- Before bed: Triphala

Thursday

- Morning: 20 oz water, anti-inflammatory drink, supplements, coffee or tea with MCT
- Take enzymes before each meal and drink 100 oz of water today.
- Breakfast: <u>Cauliflower Latkes</u>
- Lunch: <u>Chicken Caesar Salad</u>
- Dinner: <u>Mustard Lemon Chicken Legs</u>
- After dinner: One row of approved dark chocolate
- Before bed: Triphala

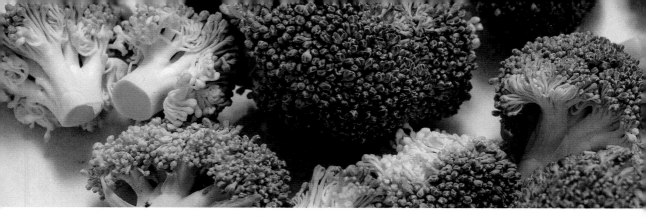

Friday (Unfasting Day)

- Morning: 20 oz water, anti-inflammatory drink, supplements, coffee or tea with MCT.
- Take enzymes before dinner and drink 100 oz water today
- Lunch: Have your metabolic boost Green drink (you can have up to 3 of these today)
- Beef, chicken, bone broth (as much as you'd like)
- 30 minutes before dinner have cacao drink
- Dinner: Beef and Broccoli
- After dinner: One row of approved dark chocolate
- Before bed: Triphala

Saturday

- Morning: 20 oz water, anti-inflammatory drink, supplements, coffee or tea with MCT
- Take enzymes before each meal and drink 100 oz of water today.
- Breakfast: Sausage and Spring Greens
- Lunch: Turkey Meatballs
- Dinner: Spicy Tuna Sushi
- After dinner: One row of approved dark chocolate and 5-6 oz red wine
- Before bed: Triphala

Week 4

Sunday

- Morning: 20 oz water, anti-inflammatory drink, supplements, coffee or tea with MCT
- Take enzymes before each meal and drink 100 oz of water today.
- Breakfast: Egg McLettuce
- Lunch: 5 Minute Keto Chili
- Dinner: Rolled Steak with Vegetables
- After dinner: One row of approved dark chocolate and 5-6 oz red wine
- Before bed: Triphala

Monday (Unfasting Day)

- Morning: 20 oz water, anti-inflammatory drink, supplements, coffee or tea with MCT.
- Take enzymes before dinner and drink 100 oz water today
- Lunch: Have your metabolic boost Green drink (you can have up to 3 of these today)
- Beef, chicken, bone broth (as much as you'd like)
- 30 minutes before dinner have cacao drink
- Dinner: Baked Herb Mahi Mahi
- After dinner: One row of approved dark chocolate
- Before bed: Triphala

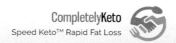

CompletelyKeto
Speed Keto™ Rapid Fat Loss

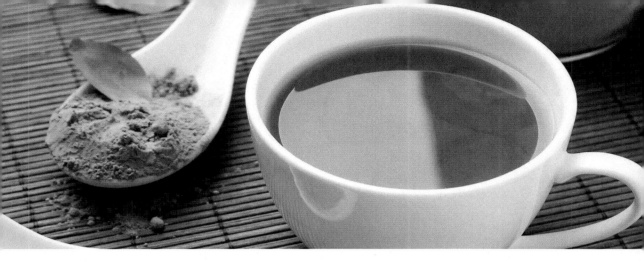

Tuesday

- Morning: 20 oz water, anti-inflammatory drink, supplements, coffee or tea with MCT
- Take enzymes before each meal and drink 100 oz of water today.
- Breakfast: Super Spicy Egg Omelet
- Lunch: Blackened Chicken Salad
- Dinner: Baked Chicken Fajitas
- After dinner: One row of approved dark chocolate
- Before bed: Triphala

Thursday

- Morning: 20 oz water, anti-inflammatory drink, supplements, coffee or tea with MCT
- Take enzymes before each meal and drink 100 oz of water today.
- Breakfast: Tuna Salad Wrap with Crepini
- Lunch: Hamburger Soup
- Dinner: Grilled Herb Tuna Skewers
- After dinner: One row of approved dark chocolate
- Before bed: Triphala

Wednesday (Unfasting Day)

- Morning: 20 oz water, anti-inflammatory drink, supplements, coffee or tea with MCT.
- Take enzymes before dinner and drink 100 oz water today
- Lunch: Have your metabolic boost Green drink (you can have up to 3 of these today)
- Beef, chicken, bone broth (as much as you'd like)
- 30 minutes before dinner have cacao drink
- Dinner: Meat Soup
- After dinner: One row of approved dark chocolate
- Before bed: Triphala

Friday (Unfasting Day)

- Morning: 20 oz water, anti-inflammatory drink, supplements, coffee or tea with MCT.
- Take enzymes before dinner and drink 100 oz water today
- Lunch: Have your metabolic boost Green drink (you can have up to 3 of these today)
- Beef, chicken, bone broth (as much as you'd like)
- 30 minutes before dinner have cacao drink
- Dinner: Chicken Pad Thai
- After dinner: One row of approved dark chocolate
- Before bed: Triphala

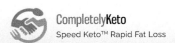

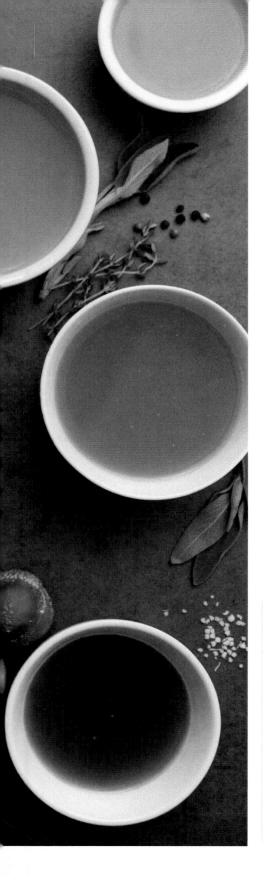

Saturday

- Morning: 20 oz water, anti-inflammatory drink, supplements, coffee or tea with MCT
- Take enzymes before each meal and drink 100 oz of water today.
- Breakfast: <u>Chocolate Tahini Shake</u>
- Lunch: <u>Ground Lamb Meat Balls</u>
- Dinner: <u>Chicken Filled with Herb Stuffing</u>
- After dinner: One row of dark chocolate and 5-6 oz red wine
- Before bed: Triphala

Week 5

Sunday

- Morning: 20 oz water, anti-inflammatory drink, supplements, coffee or tea with MCT
- Take enzymes before each meal and drink 100 oz of water today.
- Breakfast: <u>Harlan's Morning Salad</u>
- Lunch: <u>Cauliflower, Broccoli Bacon Salad</u>
- Dinner: <u>Hungarian Paprikash</u>
- After dinner: One row of approved dark chocolate and 5-6 oz red wine
- Before bed: Triphala

Monday (Unfasting Day)

- Morning: 20 oz water, anti-inflammatory drink, supplements, coffee or tea with MCT.
- Take enzymes before dinner and drink 100 oz water today
- Lunch: Have your metabolic boost Green drink (you can have up to 3 of these today)
- Beef, chicken, bone broth (as much as you'd like)
- 30 minutes before dinner have cacao drink
- Dinner: <u>Silvertip Roast</u>
- After dinner: One row of approved dark chocolate
- Before bed: Triphala

Completely**Keto**
Speed Keto™ Rapid Fat Loss

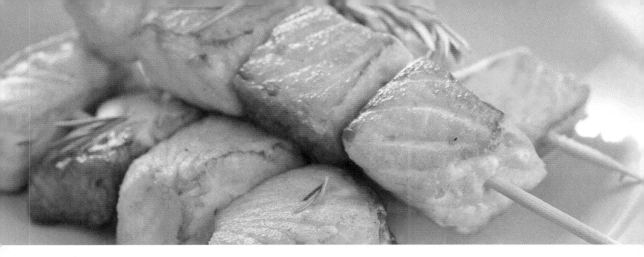

Tuesday

- Morning: 20 oz water, anti-inflammatory drink, supplements, coffee or tea with MCT
- Take enzymes before each meal and drink 100 oz of water today.
- Breakfast: Egg Salad on Bed of Spinach
- Lunch: Cucumber Tuna Roll-ups
- Dinner: Red Curry Zoodle Soup
- After dinner: One row of approved dark chocolate
- Before bed: Triphala

Wednesday (Unfasting Day)

- Morning: 20 oz water, anti-inflammatory drink, supplements, coffee or tea with MCT.
- Take enzymes before dinner and drink 100 oz water today
- Lunch: Have your metabolic boost Green drink (you can have up to 3 of these today)
- Beef, chicken, bone broth (as much as you'd like)
- 30 minutes before dinner have cacao drink
- Dinner: Kung Pao Chicken
- After dinner: One row of approved dark chocolate
- Before bed: Triphala

Thursday

- Morning: 20 oz water, anti-inflammatory drink, supplements, coffee or tea with MCT
- Take enzymes before each meal and drink 100 oz of water today.
- Breakfast: Turkey and Cucumber Roll-ups
- Lunch: Beef Zomein
- Dinner: Beef and Cauliflower Burgers
- After dinner: One row of approved dark chocolate
- Before bed: Triphala

Friday (Unfasting Day)

- Morning: 20 oz water, anti-inflammatory drink, supplements, coffee or tea with MCT.
- Take enzymes before dinner and drink 100 oz water today
- Lunch: Have your metabolic boost Green drink (you can have up to 3 of these today)
- Beef, chicken, bone broth (as much as you'd like)
- 30 minutes before dinner have cacao drink
- Dinner: Salmon Skewers
- After dinner: One row of approved dark chocolate

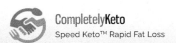

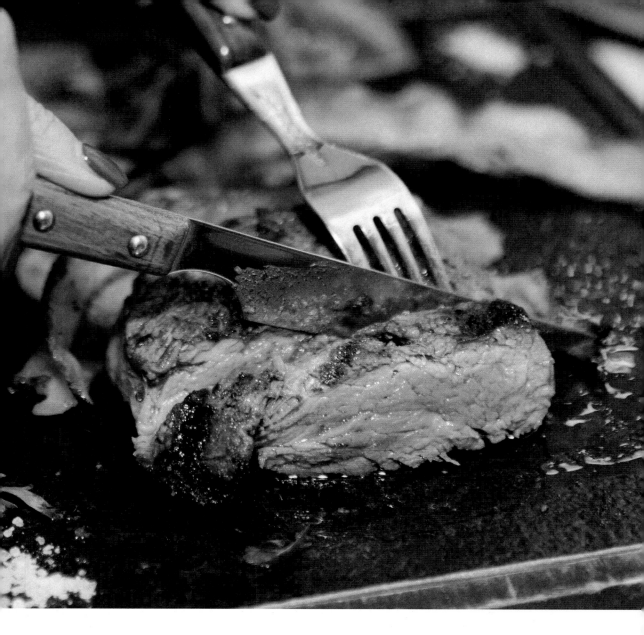

Saturday

- Morning: 20 oz water, anti-inflammatory drink, supplements, coffee or tea with MCT
- Take enzymes before each meal and drink 100 oz of water today.
- Breakfast: <u>Smoked Salmon on Bed of Arugula</u>
- Lunch: <u>Chicken Kale Spinach Salad</u>
- Dinner: <u>Pepper Steak</u>
- After dinner: One row of approved dark chocolate and 5-6 oz red wine
- Before bed: Triphala

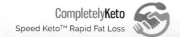

CompletelyKeto
Speed Keto™ Rapid Fat Loss

Recipes

Breakfast

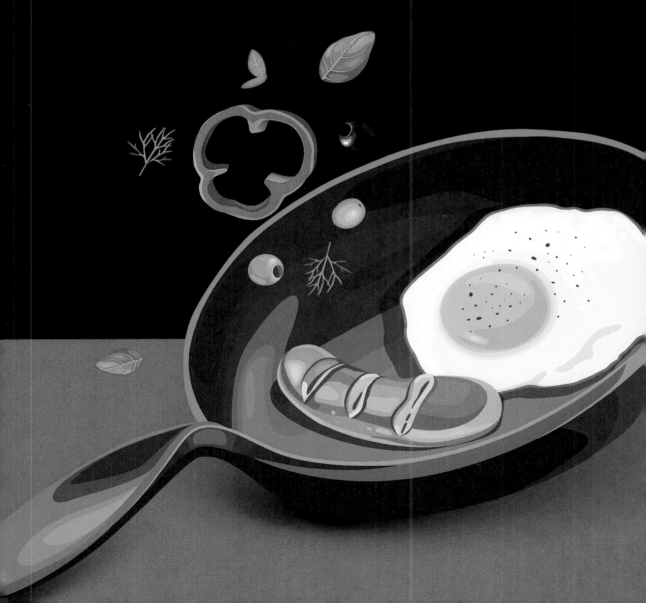

Completely Keto Strawberry Shake

Perfect for on the go and won't spike your insulin!

Servings 1

Ingredients

- 1 scoop strawberry shake
- 1.5 cup water

Instructions

1. Place shake mix and water in blender.
2. Blend until smooth.

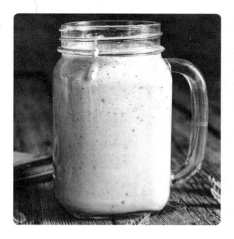

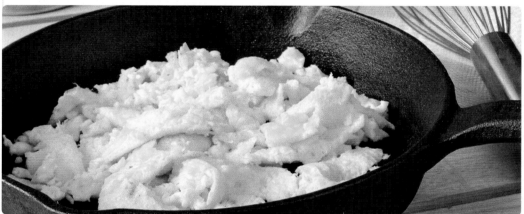

2 Scrambled Eggs (optional add hot sauce)

If you have a pair of chop sticks handy, slowly stirring the egg with chop sticks instead of tossing with a spatula gives scrambled eggs a much nicer texture.

Servings 1

Ingredients

- 2 large eggs
- 1 tsp extra virgin olive oil
- Kosher salt and fresh, cracked black pepper to taste
- Dash Franks red hot sauce (optional)

Instructions

1. Heat skillet to medium heat and add olive oil.
2. Whisk eggs well until a froth forms.
3. Pour eggs into skillet and stir until fully cooked
4. Plate and serve with salt, pepper or hot sauce.

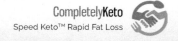

CompletelyKeto
Speed Keto™ Rapid Fat Loss

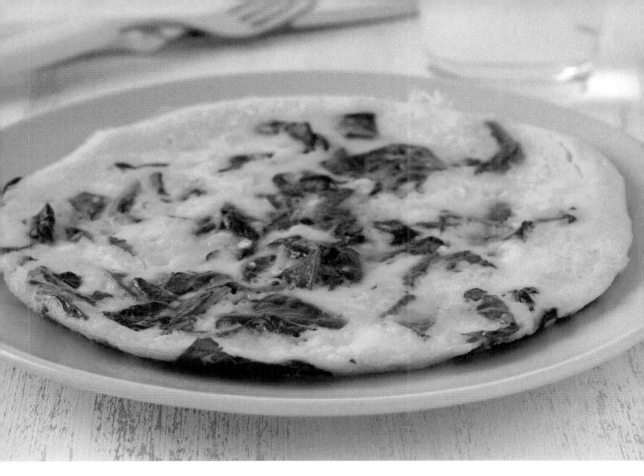

Spinach Omelet (2 eggs)

This method of cooking an omelet is only one of many. I like this one because it allows most of the egg to cook before flipping and my omelet stays nice and round.

Servings 1

Ingredients

- 2 large eggs
- 1 cup chopped baby spinach
- 1 tsp extra virgin olive oil
- Kosher salt and black pepper, as needed

Instructions

1. Chop spinach into easily mixable pieces.
2. Whisk eggs until a froth forms then add spinach to the egg and mix well.
3. Heat skillet to medium and add olive oil.
4. Pour egg mixture into skillet and push egg intermittently from the outside to the middle.
5. When egg is solid enough, flip and cook another 30 seconds to 1 minute undisturbed. Be sure not to brown the egg, reduce temperature if necessary.
6. Plate and serve with optional kosher salt and cracked black pepper.

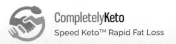

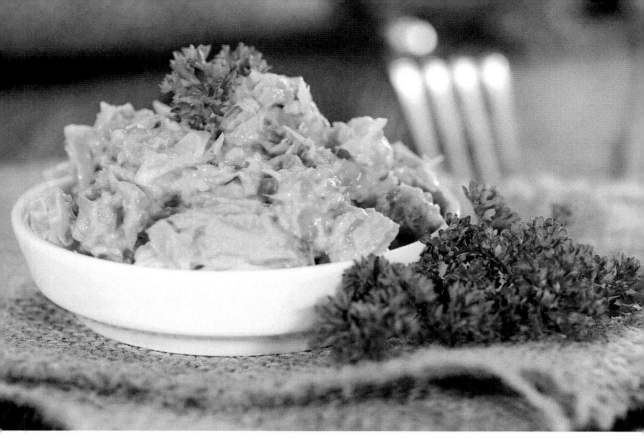

Tuna Stuffed Bell Pepper

Buying the right type of tuna will make a big difference here. The two most common types of canned tuna found in the store are chunk light and solid white albacore. Solid white albacore has a denser texture and is often an intact cut of tuna. That makes the flavor much better.

Servings 1

Ingredients

- 3.5 oz white albacore tuna in water
- 1 small green bell pepper
- 1 tbsp Primal Kitchen mayonnaise
- ½ tsp kosher salt
- 3 turns cracked black pepper
- Dash, smoked paprika

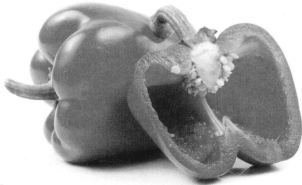

Instructions

1. Using a sharp knife, cut around the pepper stem and pull out the core. Scoop out the seeds with a spoon leaving a hollowed out pepper.
2. Mix drained tuna, spices and mayonnaise then spoon tuna mixture into the pepper.
3. Serve and enjoy.

CompletelyKeto
Speed Keto™ Rapid Fat Loss

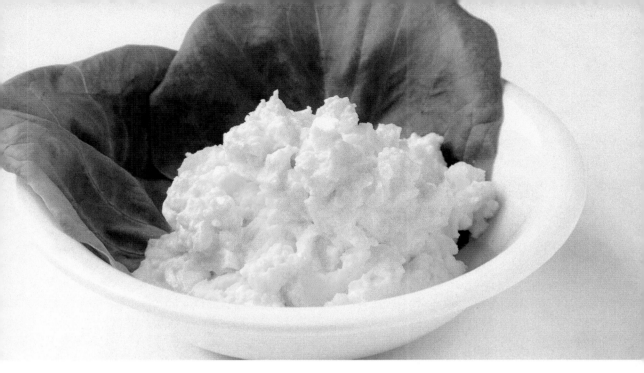

Egg Salad on a Bed of Spinach

Feel free to make a bit of extra egg salad for other breakfasts and lunches. The cooking time, water and egg cracking method is exactly the same with more eggs, just as long as they are in 1 layer in the saucepan.

Servings 1

Ingredients

- 2 hard boiled eggs
- 1 tbsp Primal Kitchen mayonnaise
- ½ tsp smoked paprika
- ½ tsp mustard powder
- ½ tsp kosher salt
- 1 cup baby spinach

Instructions

1. Place eggs in a small saucepan covered with cold water. Place on stove before turning burner on. Turn burner on high and bring to a boil.
2. Once boiling, remove saucepan from heat, cover and allow to rest covered 12-15 minutes.
3. Drain water, add a few ice cubes and cold water. Allow to rest 5 minutes.
4. Drain water, add 4 ice cubes and 2 tbsp white vinegar. Cover and shake eggs and ice in the vinegar to crack shells. Drain liquid and peel eggs.
5. Take 1 egg at a time in the palm of your hand and shred with a fork.
6. In a bowl, mix shredded egg, mayo, paprika, mustard powder and salt.
7. Plate spinach and top with egg salad.
8. Enjoy.

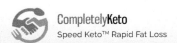

Turkey and Cucumber Roll-ups

This is a light and fresh breakfast. It's easy and quick as well when you're needing something quick in the morning.

Servings 1

Ingredients

- 3 oz thin sliced turkey
- 5 oz thin sliced cucumber with skin on.

Instructions

1. Slice cucumber into ½ inch sticks.
2. Lay turkey slices out and place cucumber sticks in the middle.
3. Roll turkey slices around cucumber.

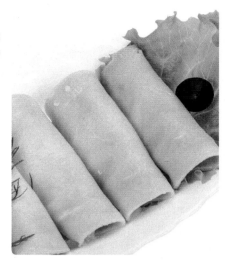

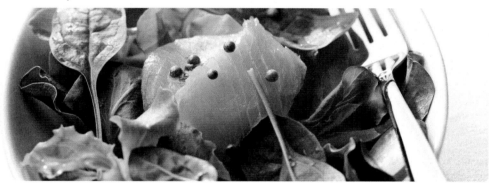

Smoked Salmon on a Bed of Arugula

Smoked salmon is already cooked so feel free to skip searing the salmon if you'd like.

Servings 1

Ingredients

- 3 oz smoked salmon, sliced thin
- 1 tbsp extra virgin olive oil
- 1 tbsp lemon juice
- 2 cups fresh arugula
- Kosher salt to taste

Instructions

1. Heat skillet to medium and add a few drops of olive oil. Sear salmon 5 seconds per side. (optional)
2. Plate arugula and place salmon on top. Drizzle with olive oil and lemon juice.
3. Serve with a sprinkle of kosher salt, and enjoy!

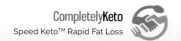

CompletelyKeto
Speed Keto™ Rapid Fat Loss

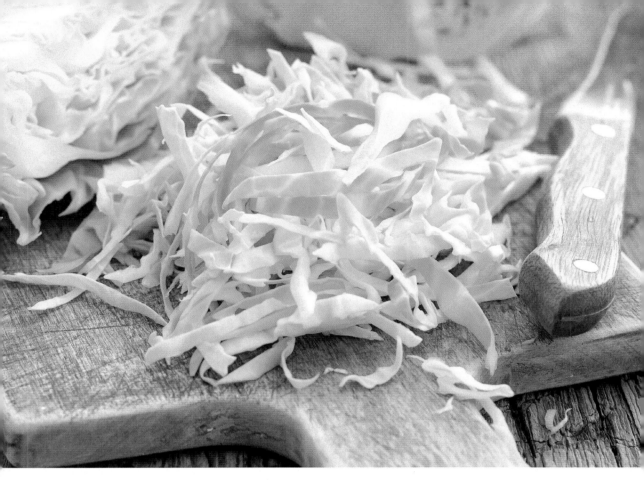

Cabbage Hash Browns

These cabbage hash browns are so delicious that you'll never want to go back to the potato version.

Servings 1

Ingredients

- 2 large eggs
- ½ tsp garlic powder
- ½ tsp kosher salt
- Freshly ground black pepper to taste
- 2 cups shredded cabbage
- ¼ small red onion, thinly sliced
- 1 tbsp extra virgin olive oil

Instructions

1. Heat skillet to medium heat and add ½ tbsp olive oil.
2. Mix all ingredients together and form pancakes.
3. Fry in batches until brown and add the rest of olive oil as needed.
4. Remove to paper towel lined plate before serving.

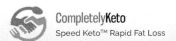

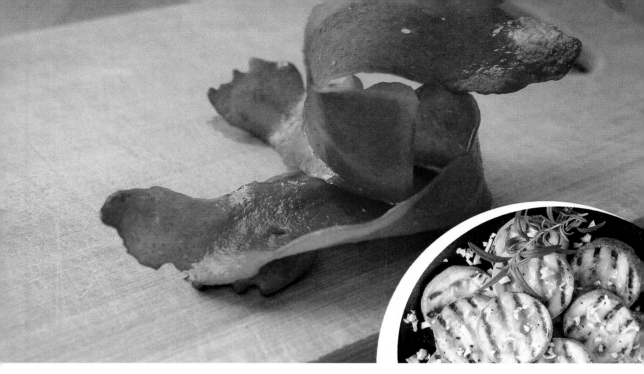

Turkey Bacon and Zucchini

Cooking zucchini can get a little tricky so keep an eye on it. Make sure keep a bit of crunch in the zucchini and not to overcook it.

Servings 1

Ingredients

- 1 medium zucchini sliced into rounds
- 1 tbsp extra virgin olive oil
- ½ tsp garlic powder
- ½ tsp onion powder
- ½ tsp kosher salt
- ½ tsp cracked black pepper
- 3 ½ oz turkey bacon (about 4 slices)

Instructions

1. Heat skillet to medium high heat and add ¼ tbsp olive oil.
2. Add bacon and fry 2-3 minutes on each side. Set aside.
3. Slice zucchini into rounds. Add the remaining olive oil to skillet and place zucchini rounds into the pan in 1 layer.
4. Sprinkle all spices over zucchini in the pan.
5. Cook 1-2 minutes and turn each slice of zucchini, cook 1 additional minute on the other side.
6. Plate zucchini and crumble turkey bacon on top.
7. Serve and enjoy!

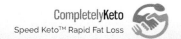

CompletelyKeto
Speed Keto™ Rapid Fat Loss

Sausage and Spring Greens

Feel free to use any type of sugar free turkey or chicken sausage you like; links, patties or ground sausage. For this recipe we like ground sausage.

Servings 1

Ingredients

- 3 oz turkey or chicken sausage
- ½ tsp extra virgin olive oil
- 1 cup spring mix
- 1 tsp lemon juice
- Dash of paprika

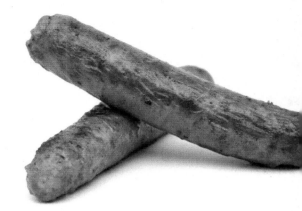

Instructions

1. Heat a skillet to medium high heat and add olive oil.
2. Add ground sausage to pan and brown while breaking apart. About 3 minutes.
3. Plate spring mix and add sausage to the top.
4. Drizzle lemon juice over top and sprinkle with paprika.
5. Serve and enjoy.

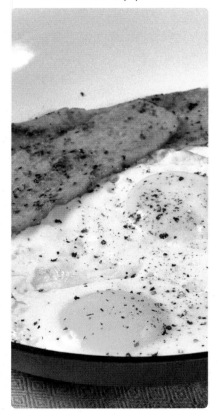

Bacon and Egg

Cook your egg however you like. If you like a sunny side up egg, just set your heat lower so you don't brown the bottom while the top whites have a chance to cook.

Servings 1

Ingredients

- Turkey bacon 3.5 oz
- 1 sunny side up egg
- 1 tsp extra virgin olive oil

Instructions

1. Heat skillet to medium high heat and add ½ tsp olive oil.
2. Add bacon and fry 2 minutes per side, remove and set aside.
3. Add the remaining olive oil to pan and crack egg into the pan.
4. Reduce heat to medium low to medium and cook egg slowly until white is cooked and yolk is still runny. About 3-4 minutes.
5. Plate with turkey bacon and serve.

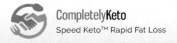

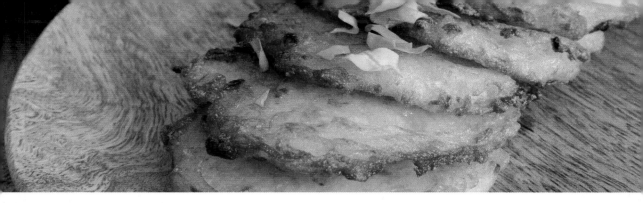

Cauliflower Latkes

These do need a bit more oil than some of our other recipes in order to cook well. If you need to add a bit to this recipe that is fine.

They freeze well.

Servings 2

Ingredients

- 24 oz cauliflower rice
- 1 small red onion
- 4 large eggs beaten well
- 1 tsp Xanthan Gum
- 1 tbsp sea salt
- 1/2 tsp black pepper
- 4 tbsp extra virgin olive oil for frying

Instructions

1. Using fresh or frozen riced cauliflower, heat up a skillet with some oil on the bottom and add riced cauliflower to the skillet.
2. Sauté until well cooked, stirring occasionally for about 5 -7 minutes on medium- low and set aside.
3. Cut the onion into 6 pieces and place in food processor, leaving the onions smooth and having no large pieces.
4. Add onion to the cooked cauliflower and mix well.
5. In a bowl whisk 4 eggs together with a beater until well beaten.
6. Add the cooked, riced cauliflower and onion mix to the bowl and stir.
7. Add the salt, pepper and xanthan gum and mix well.
8. In an electric fryer or deep skillet heat up oil until bubbling slightly.
9. Using an ice cream scoop or a measuring cup of ¼ cup size drop the mixture into the oil, never frying too many too closely.
10. Leave space in between, as they will spread in size.
11. Fry until golden in color.
12. Remove and place onto a prepared plate of paper towels to drain excess oil.
13. Serve on a plate and enjoy.

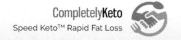
CompletelyKeto
Speed Keto™ Rapid Fat Loss

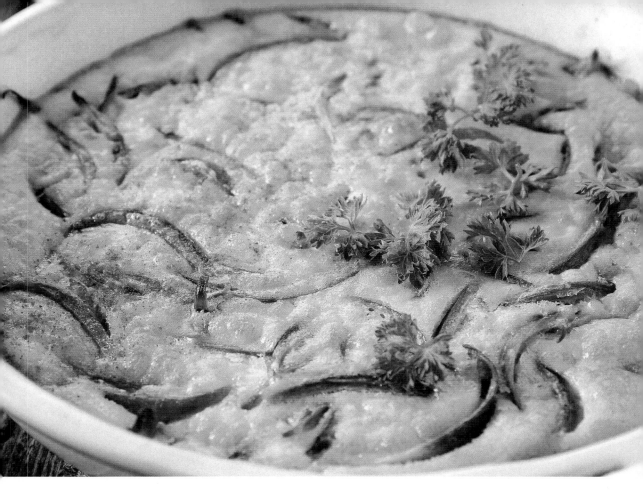

Red Onion Omelet

Onions add the perfect bite to fluffy eggs in this omelet recipe.

Servings 1

Ingredients

- 2 eggs
- ¼ diced small red onion
- ½ tsp extra virgin olive oil

Instructions

1. Whisk eggs well until a froth begins to form.
2. Dice onion finely.
3. Heat skillet to medium heat and add olive oil.
4. Mix onion into egg mixture.
5. Pour egg mixture into pan and push egg from the outer corners in, allowing the uncooked egg to flow into the bare parts of the pan.
6. When egg is solid enough, flip and continue to cook for up to 1 minute, undisturbed.
7. Plate and serve.

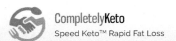

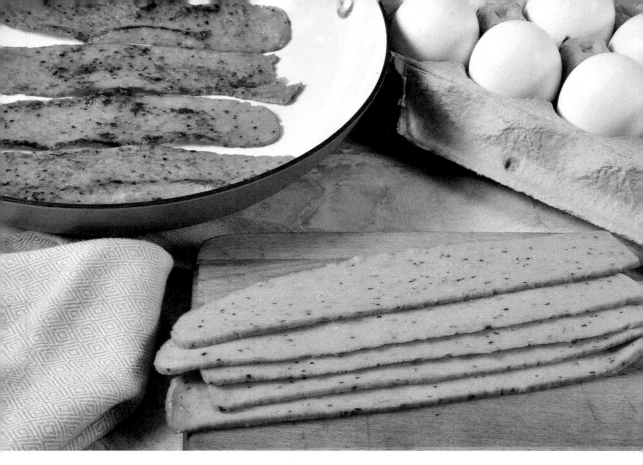

Egg McLettuce

This recipe calls for a sunny side up egg, but feel free to cook the egg however you like to wrap in the lettuce.

Servings 1

Ingredients

- 2 slices Turkey Bacon
- 1 sunny side up egg
- 2 slices romaine lettuce
- 1 tsp extra virgin olive oil

Instructions

1. Heat skillet to medium high heat, add ½ tsp olive oil.
2. Add bacon and cook 2 minutes per side or until crispy. Set aside.
3. Rinse any residue from pan and reduce heat to just below medium. Add ½ tsp olive oil and crack egg into pan. Cook 2-3 minutes, slowly so that the white is cooked and the yolk is left runny.
4. Add spices of choice.
5. Serve bacon and egg on romaine leaves and enjoy.

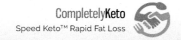

CompletelyKeto
Speed Keto™ Rapid Fat Loss

Lox Eggs and Onion

Be sure to look at ingredients and nutrition information when buying your smoked salmon. Sometimes they will smoke with sugar. You want to find a sugar free smoked salmon.

Servings 1

Ingredients

- 1 egg
- ¼ red onion, sliced thin
- 3 oz smoked salmon

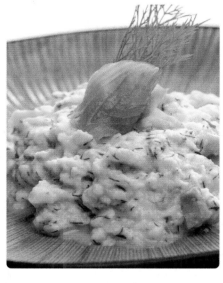

Instructions

1. Heat skillet to medium heat and add ½ tsp olive oil.
2. Scramble egg with onion and smoked salmon at the same time. Cook while stirring about 1-2 minutes.
3. Plate and serve with an optional vegetable.

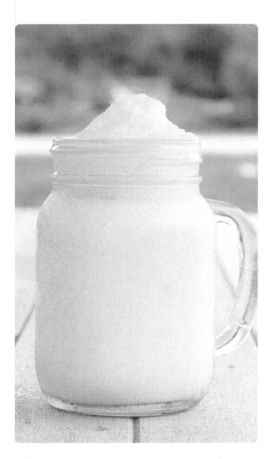

Chana's Special Tahini Shake

This shake is full of nutrients and is quick and delicious.

Servings 1

Ingredients

- 1/2 cup full fat coconut cream
- 2 tbsp tahini (comes in glass jars).
- 1/8 tsp cinnamon
- 8-12 ice cubes
- 1-2 drops Sweet leaf stevia

Instructions

1. Add all ingredients to your blender.
2. Beat until creamy.
3. Pour into glass and serve.

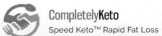

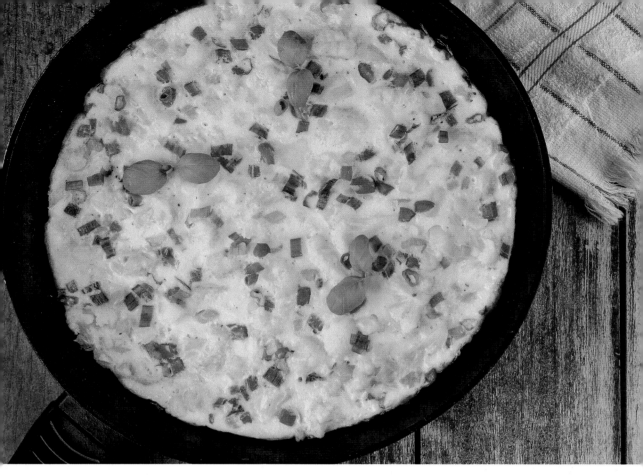

Super Spicy Egg Omelet

This omelet lives up to its name. Feel free to skip the hot sauce if you'd like it a bit less spicy.

Servings 2

Ingredients

- 2 eggs, scrambled
- 2 tbsp spicy salsa or pico de gallo
- Hot sauce to taste
- 5 cucumber slices
- 1 tsp extra virgin olive oil

Instructions

1. Heat skillet to medium heat and add olive oil.
2. Whisk eggs and add salsa to egg mixture.
3. Pour egg and salsa mixture into the hot pan.
4. Push egg to the middle with a spatula allowing the uncooked egg to flow onto the space, repeat on the other side. When egg is cooked enough to stay together, flip and cook 30 seconds to 1 minute more.
5. Plate and serve with a dash of hot sauce and sliced cucumbers on the side.

CompletelyKeto
Speed Keto™ Rapid Fat Loss

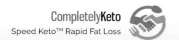

Tuna Salad Wrap

The type of canned tuna used in this recipe makes all the difference. The solid white albacore tuna has a much nicer texture than chunk light.

Servings 1

Ingredients

- 3 1/2 oz of canned solid white albacore tuna in water
- 2 tbsp Primal Kitchen mayo
- 1 stalk celery, diced
- ½ tsp kosher salt
- Black pepper to taste
- 1 Crepini Cauliflower Wrap

Instructions

1. Drain water from tuna.
2. Mix all ingredients together.
3. Serve in Crepini Cauliflower wrap.

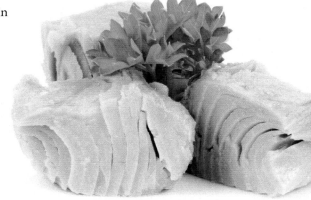

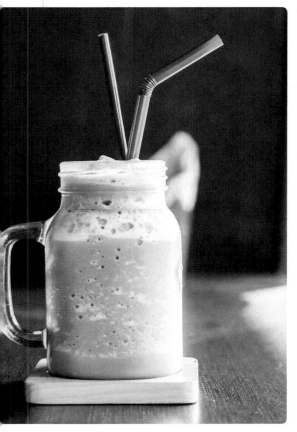

Chocolate Tahini Shake

This shake has everything you need to stay fueled until lunch.

Servings 1

Ingredients

- 1/2 cup full fat coconut cream
- 1 tsp approved cocoa powder
- 2 tbsp tahini (comes in glass jars).
- 1/8 tsp cinnamon
- 8-12 ice cubes
- 1-2 drops Sweet leaf stevia

Instructions

1. Add all ingredients to your blender.
2. Beat until creamy.
3. Add straw.

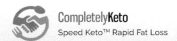

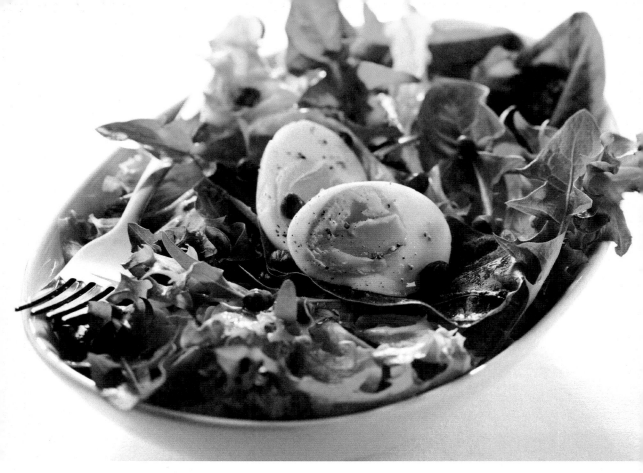

Harlan's Morning Salad

This salad is packed with nutritious leafy greens and filling hard boiled eggs. Light, fresh and delicious.

Servings 1

Ingredients

- 2 hardboiled eggs, cut in quarters
- 1 handful chopped kale
- 1 handful spinach
- ½ English cucumber, sliced
- Slivers of fresh fennel, sliced very thin (good for digestion)
- Sprinkle some alfalfa sprouts on salad
- 2 or 3 dandelion greens, chopped small
- 2 tbsp tahini dressing

Instructions

1. Plate all salad greens and vegetables.
2. Slice hard boiled eggs and add to plate.
3. Top with tahini dressing

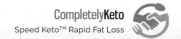

CompletelyKeto
Speed Keto™ Rapid Fat Loss

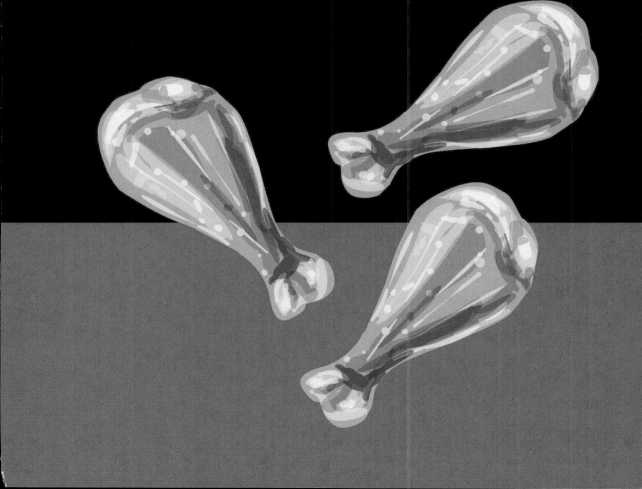

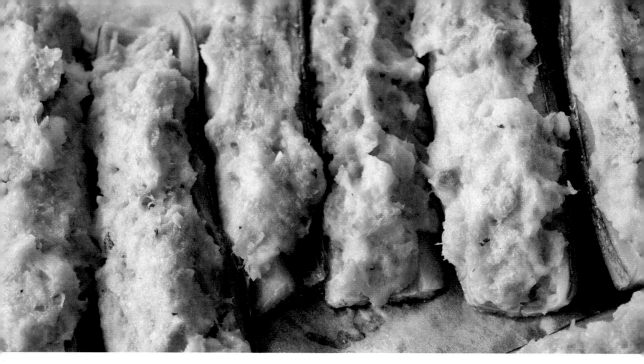

Tuna on a Log

These are an amazing treat. Be sure to brown your zucchini but don't let it get too mushy. They should still be nice and firm to hold the tuna.

Servings 1

Ingredients

- 1 medium zucchini
- 1 garlic clove, minced
- 3 ½ oz tuna (or salmon) in a can, in water
- 1 tbsp Primal Kitchen Mayonnaise
- 1 tsp celery salt
- Black pepper to taste
- 2 sprigs fresh parsley
- 1 tsp extra virgin olive oil

Instructions

1. Cut zucchini in half, lengthwise. Remove all seeds carefully not to break the zucchini, using a small spoon or melon scooper.
2. Heat skillet to medium heat and add olive oil.
3. Place zucchini halves into the pan open side up.
4. Cook 3-5 minutes. Take care not to let zucchini get too soft.
5. In a medium sized bowl, add tuna or salmon, celery salt, black pepper, garlic and mayo. Mix well.
6. Remove zucchini from heat and spoon tuna or salmon mix into the logs.
7. Garnish with parsley and serve.

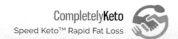

CompletelyKeto
Speed Keto™ Rapid Fat Loss

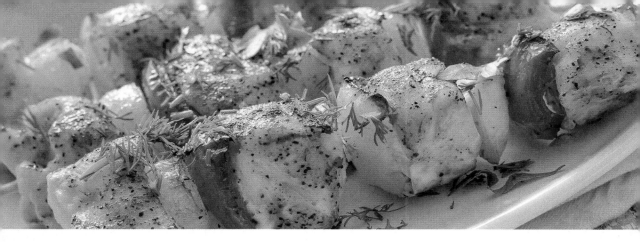

Chicken and Vegetable Kebabs

These skewers can be made easily in the oven or on the grill. We have provided you with a few different cooking methods to make this delicious recipe.

Servings 1

Ingredients

- 3 ½ oz chicken breast, cubed
- 1 tbsp fresh lemon juice
- 2 tbsp extra virgin olive oil
- 2 tbsp wheat free tamari
- 1 large garlic clove, crushed
- 1 lemons zest
- ¼ medium red onion
- ½ large bell pepper

Instructions

Grill:

1. Cut the onions, peppers, and chicken into cubes and place in three separate bowls.
2. Mix all the other ingredients in a blender or food processor. Pour over the chicken bowl.
3. Mix the marinade well with the chicken cubes, so it's totally enveloped in marinade. Let marinate for at least 3 hours in the fridge.
4. Pierce the chicken, onion and pepper cubes intermittently as you see fit on to wooden sticks.
5. Grill all the skewers until the chicken is 165° internally. About 10-15 minutes over direct heat or 20-25 minutes over indirect heat.

Oven:

1. Pre-heat the oven to 500°F and heat a grill pan over high heat for 4-5 minutes.
2. Place the chicken skewers on the pan and grill for 2-3 minutes, then flip and grill for another 2 minutes. Transfer pan to the oven and cook for another 5 minutes.
3. For the baking option without a grill pan
4. Place the kebabs on a baking sheet and bake at 500°F for 10-12 minutes.

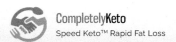

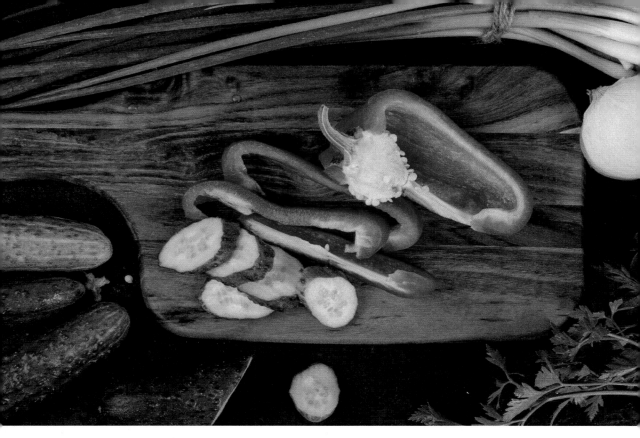

Greek Salad

This salad is a lot like the one you'll see at a Greek restaurant. It has no lettuce to allow the crunch and flavors of the delicious vegetables shine through.

Servings 1

Ingredients

- ½ green bell pepper, diced
- ½ cucumber, sliced
- ½ tsp garlic powder
- 1 tbsp Primal Kitchen mayonnaise
- 1 tbsp extra virgin olive oil
- 2 tbsp apple cider vinegar
- ½ red onion, diced
- ½ tsp Pink Himalayan Salt
- 5 black olives
- ½ tsp black pepper

Instructions

1. Mix the mayo, olive oil, vinegar and spices in a small bowl.
2. Chop all vegetables into cubes and transfer to salad bowl.
3. Pour desired amount of mayo mix over the salad and toss until fully coated and combined.

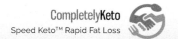

CompletelyKeto
Speed Keto™ Rapid Fat Loss

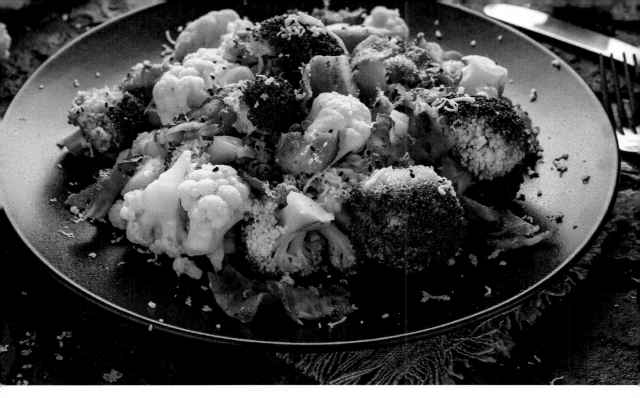

Cauliflower, Broccoli and Bacon Salad

Since we can now buy pre-washed salad greens and bacon that is already cooked, making noon-time salads is quick and easy. You can whip this salad together when lunch time rolls around or prepare it in the morning to take to work. This salad holds up well when dressed in the morning and consumed at noon.

Servings 2

Ingredients

- 1 cup cauliflower florets
- 1 cup broccoli florets
- 3 turkey bacon strips, cooked and crumbled
- ½ red onion thinly slices (about ¼ C)
- 3 tbsp primal kitchen mayonnaise
- 2 tsp fresh lemon (or lime) juice
- 1 tsp dried tarragon (or 1 tbsp fresh leaves)
- 2 cups baby spinach leaves
- Grinding of pink Himalayan salt and black peppercorns, to taste

Instructions

1. Pulse cauliflower and broccoli florets in a food processor until small chunks form. Toss with crumbled turkey bacon and red onion.
2. To make a dressing whisk the mayonnaise, lemon juice and tarragon. Add to salad and toss.
3. Divide spinach and onion between 2 salad plates and arrange the cauliflower/broccoli and bacon salad on top. Season with salt and pepper to taste. Serve immediately.

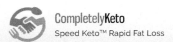

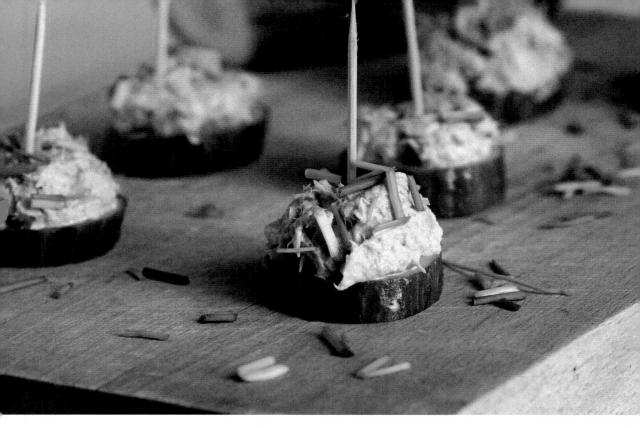

Cucumber and Tuna Roll-ups

Keeping canned tuna on hand for a quick lunch is always a good idea. These easy-to-assemble pinwheel roll-ups are elegant and at the same time, economical and practical.

Servings 2

Ingredients

- 2 English cucumber
- 1 can solid white albacore tuna in water
- ¼ red onion, minced
- 4 tbsp Primal Kitchen mayonnaise, divided
- 1 tbsp fresh lemon juice
- Hot sauce, to taste (no sugar)

Instructions

1. Leave the green skin on the cucumbers. Use a vegetable peeler to make long thin cucumber slices. Make them as thin as possible so they will be flexible when it's time to roll them up.
2. Mix tuna and red onion with 2 tbsp of mayonnaise.
3. Whisk lemon juice and hot sauce with the remaining mayonnaise to make a dressing.
4. Spread tuna onto the full length of each cucumber slice. Roll the cucumber into a pinwheel. Secure with a toothpick if necessary.
5. Repeat until all the ingredients have been used.

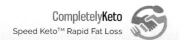

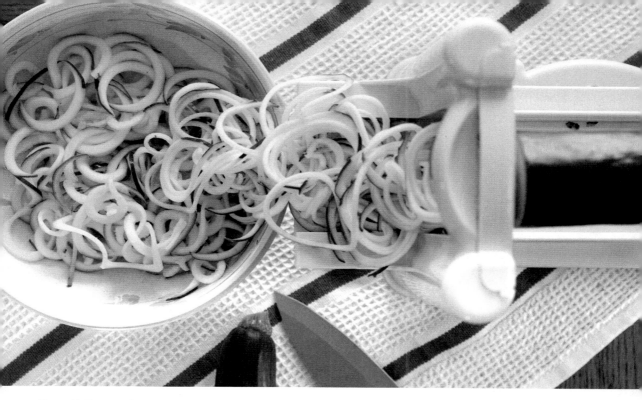

Beef Zomein

This is great for weekends so you can have leftovers. Spice it up as much as you like.

Servings 4

Ingredients

- 1 lb beef, cut into small thin pieces such as flank steak or similar
- 10 string beans, cut into 1/4 pieces
- 2 chili peppers, chopped into thin slices
- 3 cloves garlic, minced
- 3 tbsp wheat free tamari sauce
- 3 tbsp extra virgin olive oil
- 2 large zucchinis, made into zoodles using Spiralizer
- 1 tsp pink Himalayan Salt
- 2 tbsp Pinot Noir (optional)

Instructions

1. Using your spiralizer, make the zucchinis into a big bowl of zoodles and set aside.
2. Heat a large skillet on medium heat and add extra virgin olive oil.
3. Toss in pieces of beef, string beans, garlic, tamari and salt. Stir continuously until beef is cooked through. About 3 minutes.
4. Pour the 2 tbsp of wine in and deglaze stirring for 30 seconds.
5. Add the zoodles to mixture and toss to coat well. Cover and steam 1 minute.
6. Serve and enjoy.

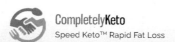

CompletelyKeto
Speed Keto™ Rapid Fat Loss

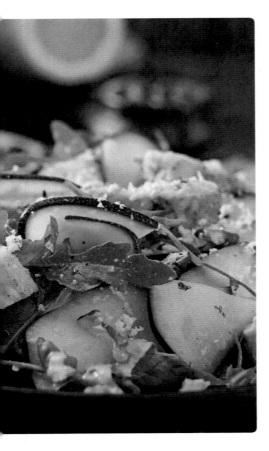

Chicken Kale Spinach Salad

The two types of greens in this salad provide an amazing contrast in texture. The crunchy kale and delicate spinach make this a perfect, light and fresh dish.

Servings 1

Ingredients

- 3 ½ oz chicken breast
- ½ oz kale
- 2 oz baby spinach
- ¼ small red onion, sliced thin
- ¼ cucumber, sliced in quarter chunks
- 2 scallions, diced

Instructions

1. Preheat oven to 425 degrees.
2. Line a baking pan with parchment paper and bake chicken for about 15 minutes.
3. Cut baked chicken into strips and add into a large bowl with all the rest of the ingredients.
4. Top with basil salad dressing and toss well.
5. Store the rest of the dressing for future use.

Basil Dressing

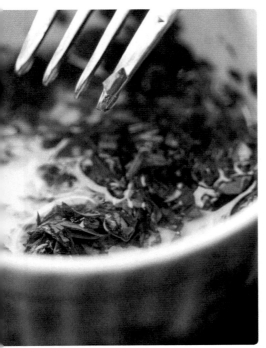

Ingredients

- 1 tbsp lemon juice
- 1 tbsp extra virgin olive oil
- 1 tbsp apple cider vinegar
- 1 garlic cloves, minced
- 5 leaves fresh basil
- 1 tsp Pink Himalayan Salt
- 1 tsp black pepper

Instructions

1. Simply blend the ingredients to the texture of your preference.
2. Enjoy!

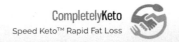

CompletelyKeto
Speed Keto™ Rapid Fat Loss

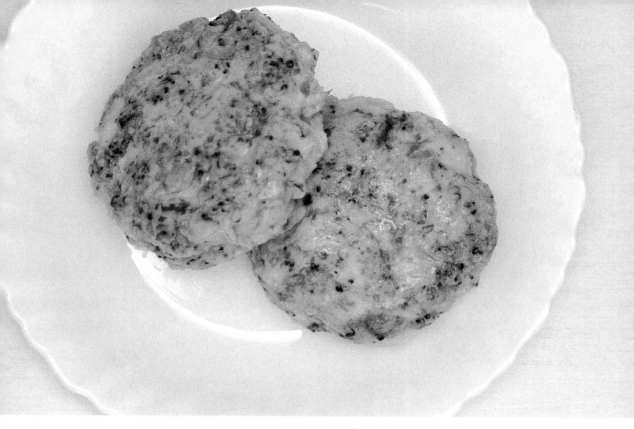

Turkey Zucchini Burgers

In this recipe, instead of having turkey burgers with a veggie on the side, we have all the ingredients together for a veggie and meat burger.

Servings 4

Ingredients

- 1 lb ground turkey
- ¼ tsp Pink Himalayan Salt
- ¼ tsp black pepper
- 1 garlic clove, minced
- ¼ tsp ground ginger
- 1 small red onion, diced
- 1 tbsp wheat free tamari sauce
- 1 cup zucchini, shredded

Instructions

1. Set oven to 375 degrees.
2. Prep a baking pan with a parchment paper.
3. Mix all ingredients in a bowl together well and make patties.
4. Bake the patties in the oven for about 18 minutes then flip and continue baking for 5-10 minutes.
5. Serve and enjoy.

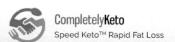

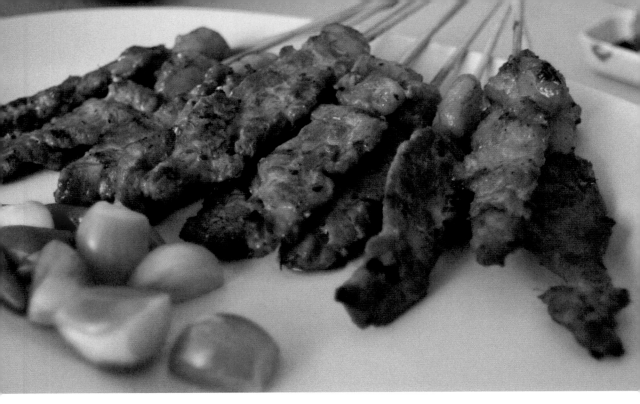

Beef Satay

These are easy to make and easy to eat. They taste amazing with the smoky flavors from the grill. Wheat free tamari tastes great for dipping.

Servings 4

Ingredients

- 1 lb ground beef
- 1 tbsp wheat free tamari sauce
- 1 tbsp minced garlic
- 1 tbsp minced ginger
- ¼ red onion, diced
- ½ tsp dried basil
- ½ tsp Chinese 5 spice
- 2 tbsp extra virgin olive oil

Instructions

1. Combine all ingredients (except the oil) and mix well using clean hands.
2. Form meat around small wooden skewers. Brush with olive oil.
3. Pre-heat grill to medium high heat.
4. Grill skewers for 3 minutes on one side and flip.
5. Continue to grill for a few more minutes or until the internal temperature reaches 165 F.
6. Serve skewers with any RFL approved sauce of choice on the side.

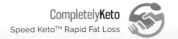
CompletelyKeto
Speed Keto™ Rapid Fat Loss

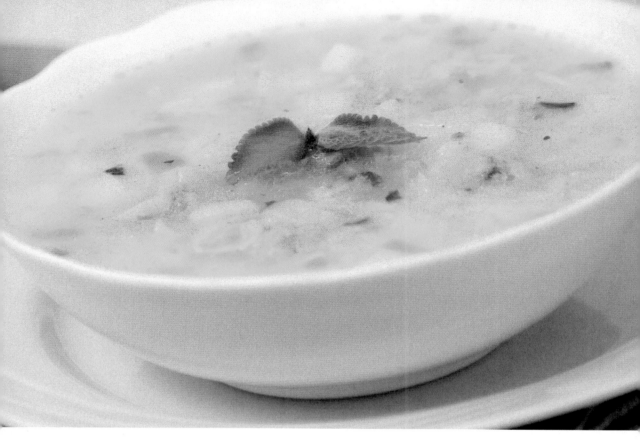

Chicken and Rice Soup

There's nothing better than chicken soup. It's good for the mind and body. This lunch will be easy because you'll be using leftover chicken.

Servings 1

Ingredients

- ½ cup diced cooked chicken (leftovers)
- ½ small red onion
- ½ tbsp extra virgin olive oil
- ½ tsp thyme
- 1 quart homemade or purchased chicken broth
- 1 cup riced cauliflower
- ¼ cup minced Parsley (curly not Italian)

Instructions

1. Heat skillet to medium heat and add olive oil.
2. Simmer onion in olive oil until soft about 2 minutes.
3. Stir in cooked chicken and spices.
4. Add cauliflower and chicken broth. Stir for 5-8 minutes until soup is hot.
5. Serve and enjoy.

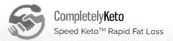

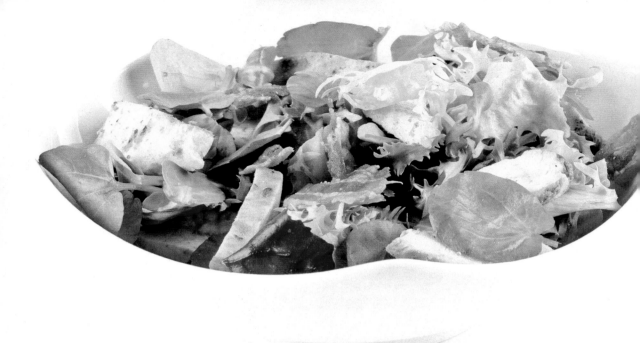

Chicken Caesar Salad

Traditionally Caesar dressing does include anchovies but we have not included them in this recipe. If you'd like to add a bit into the dressing mixture, that's perfectly fine. Be sure to rinse your vegetables well under cold water before chopping.

Servings 1

Ingredients

- 1 turkey bacon strip
- 1 cup of Romaine lettuce, shredded
- ½ cup arugula
- 2 tsp lemon juice
- ½ tbsp mustard
- 2 tbsp Primal Kitchen mayo
- 3 oz cooked chicken breast
- Salt and pepper to taste

Instructions

1. Heat skillet to medium high and add turkey bacon. Fry turkey bacon strip until done, about 3 minutes.
2. Place torn romaine and arugula in large bowl.
3. Mix lemon juice, mustard and mayo.
4. Add salt and pepper to your taste.
5. Drizzle dressing on top of romaine mix.
6. Top with cooked chicken and bacon crumbles.

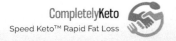

CompletelyKeto
Speed Keto™ Rapid Fat Loss

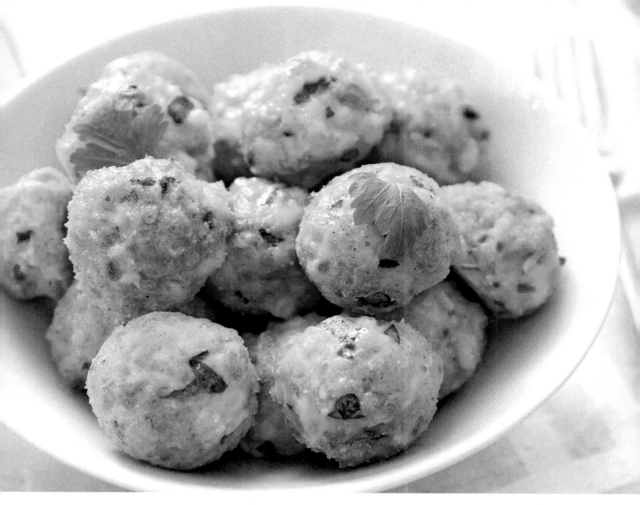

Turkey Meatballs

This recipe will have leftovers. Use for dinner or another lunch. If you want just for one person, start with 4 oz of ground turkey.

Servings 4

Ingredients

- 1 lb ground turkey
- ¼ cup minced parsley
- 1 tbsp minced garlic
- 1 tbsp wheat free tamari sauce
- 2 tbsp approved ketchup
- 1 tbsp extra virgin olive oil

Instructions

1. Heat skillet to medium low and add olive oil.
2. Mix all ingredients together in a bowl and form meatballs with your hands.
3. Fry them in pan until well cooked on all sides, about 12-15 minutes, turning each meatball intermittently.

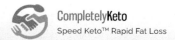

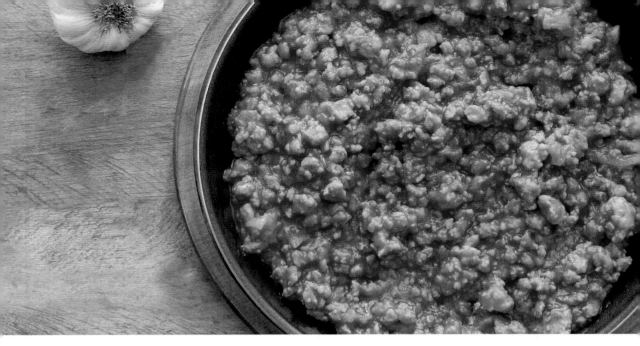

5 Minute Keto Chili

This is great for weekends so you can have leftovers. Spice it up as much as you like. In this recipe we are using ground chicken, but beef or turkey work well also.

Servings 4

1 tbsp extra virgin olive oil

- ½ small red onion
- 1 tbsp minced garlic
- 1 lb ground beef, turkey, or chicken
- ½ tbsp chili powder
- ½ tbsp smoked paprika
- ½ tsp ground cumin
- 3 tsp chipotle
- Salt and black pepper to taste
- 1 ½ cups beef broth
- 2 cups riced cauliflower
- 2 tbsp approved ketchup

Instructions

1. Heat skillet to medium heat and add olive oil.
2. Brown onions in olive oil, then add ground beef and spices. Break apart while cooking and cook through.
3. Add beef broth and stir.
4. Add riced cauliflower and ketchup.
5. Simmer on top of stove for 1 hour, stirring intermittently.
6. Serve hot and enjoy.

CompletelyKeto
Speed Keto™ Rapid Fat Loss

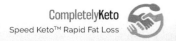

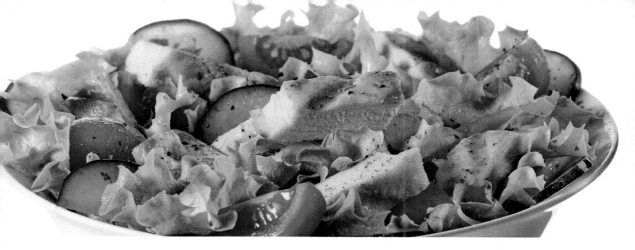

Blackened Chicken Salad

This recipe makes enough for the whole family to enjoy a light and refreshing chicken salad.

Servings 6

Ingredients

Chicken:

- 24 oz chicken; 6 - 4 oz pieces of white or dark chicken
- 1 tbsp extra virgin olive oil
- 3 tsp poultry seasoning

Salad

- 1 head lettuce or a bag of spring greens
- 1 long English cucumber, sliced thin
- 1 small red onion, chopped into small cubes
- 1 red bell pepper, diced
- 8 cherry tomatoes, halved (after round 1, only)

Dressing:

- 4 tbsp extra virgin olive oil
- 1 fresh lemon juice only
- 1 tsp pink Himalayan Salt
- 1 pinch ground black pepper

Instructions

1. Sprinkle each piece of chicken with poultry seasoning on both sides evenly.
2. Preheat oven to 350° F and grease a baking pan with extra virgin olive oil .
3. Place chicken in preheated oven and cook 35-40 minutes.
4. Remove and set aside.
5. Mix salad dressing in a jar or small bowl.
6. Plate salad greens and vegetables, then place tenderized and blackened chicken on top and pour dressing over.
7. Enjoy!

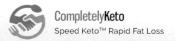

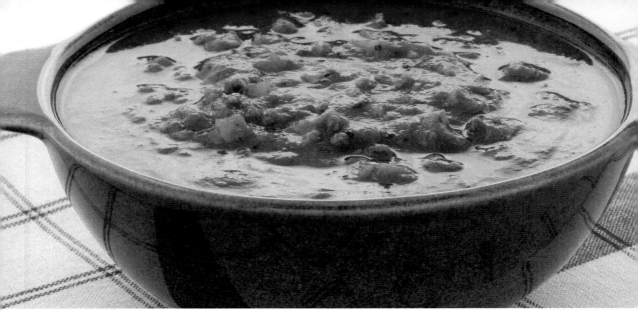

Hamburger Soup

This soup is hearty and delicious. Perfect on a chilly afternoon.

Servings 4

Ingredients

- 3 small red onions, diced
- 1 tsp xanthan gum, mixed with 3 tsp of water
- 10 cups water
- 2 tsp pink Himalayan Salt
- 1 tsp black pepper
- ½ cup Pinot Noir (optional)
- 2 tbsp onion powder
- 1 tbsp garlic powder
- 1 pound ground beef

Instructions

1. Heat skillet to medium high heat.
2. Add beef and brown while breaking apart. When done add to a large pot.
3. Reduce heat to medium and add onions to the fat in the pan leftover from cooking the hamburger meat. Saute for about 4 minutes until they start to turn a golden brown. Transfer onions to the pot with the beef.
4. Mix the teaspoons of xanthan gum and water in a bowl and add to the pot.
5. Add all the rest of the ingredients to the pot including the cups of water together and mix well.
6. Place pot on stove top on medium high heat.
7. Let the soup reach a boil, then reduce to medium low and cook for 2 hours.
8. Serve and enjoy.

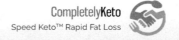

CompletelyKeto
Speed Keto™ Rapid Fat Loss

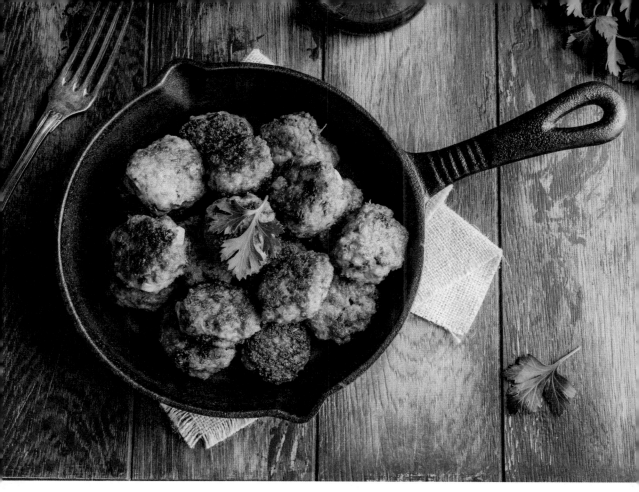

Ground Lamb Balls

Enjoy these with a salad on the side.

Servings 4

Ingredients

- 1 ½ lb ground lamb
- 3 tbsp parsley chopped
- 1 tsp pink Himalayan Salt
- 4 garlic cloves, grated
- ½ cup red onion, grated
- ½ tsp black pepper
- 2 egg whites

Instructions

1. Preheat oven to 375°F.
2. Mix all ingredients together well. Spoon them into ball shaped size.
3. Grease a baking pan and line with parchment paper. Bake for around 25 minutes.
4. Serve and enjoy.

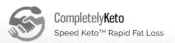

CompletelyKeto
Speed Keto™ Rapid Fat Loss

Recipes
—
Dinner

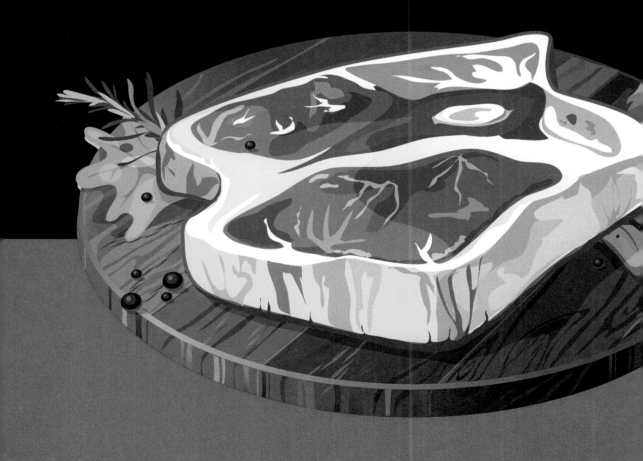

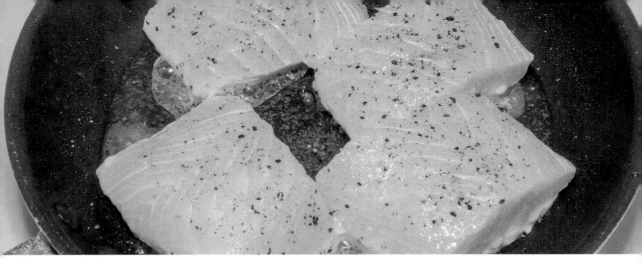

Baked Herb Mahi Mahi with Balsamic Glaze

This light fish pairs perfectly with the rich balsamic glaze. When simmering the vinegar down be sure to keep stirring so that it forms a uniform and thick consistency.

Servings 4

Ingredients

- 4 mahi mahi fillets, 3-4 oz each
- Pink Himalayan Salt to taste
- Cracked black pepper to taste
- 2 tbsp parsley chopped
- 2 tbsp extra virgin olive oil
- 2 tbsp basil
- 2 tbsp garlic, minced
- 2 tbsp oregano
- 2 tbsp capers
- 2 tbsp lemon juice

Balsamic Glaze:

- 1 cup balsamic vinegar
- Simmer on low heat in a saucepan until reduced to 1/3 of its original size

Instructions

1. Set oven to 425 degrees.
2. Season the fish with salt and pepper.
3. Mix all other ingredients in a bowl and set aside.
4. Heat an oven safe skillet to medium high heat and grease with olive oil.
5. Add fish to pan and cook 3-4 minutes to form a nice crust on one side.
6. Carefully flip fish and transfer pan to the middle rack of the oven.
7. Cook in oven about 5-6 minutes until center is cooked through.
8. Remove from oven and drizzle the glaze over.

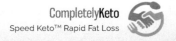

CompletelyKeto
Speed Keto™ Rapid Fat Loss

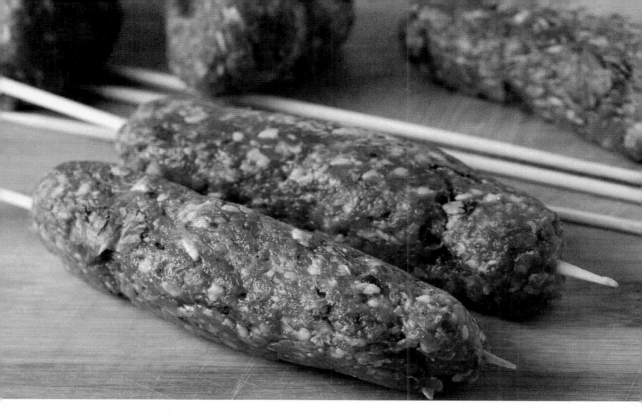

Beef Skewers

When grilling with wooden skewers, soak them in water for a minimum of 10 minutes so they don't burn on the heat while cooking.

Servings 6

Ingredients

- Skewers
- ¼ tsp black pepper
- ¼ tsp turmeric
- 1 tsp pink Himalayan Salt
- 1 small red onion, grated
- 1 ½ lbs ground beef
- ¼ tsp cumin, ground

Instructions

1. Mix all the ingredients well in a bowl by kneading it with your hands until fully combined.
2. Cover and let it sit in the fridge for a while to mix the flavors together.
3. Take a handful of the beef mix and form around the skewer to resemble a sausage with the skewer in the middle.
4. Repeat with all the rest of the beef and skewers.
5. Preheat a grill or a prepped greased grill pan. Place kebabs onto the heat and keep turning them until they are fully cooked, about 5 minutes.

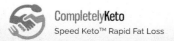

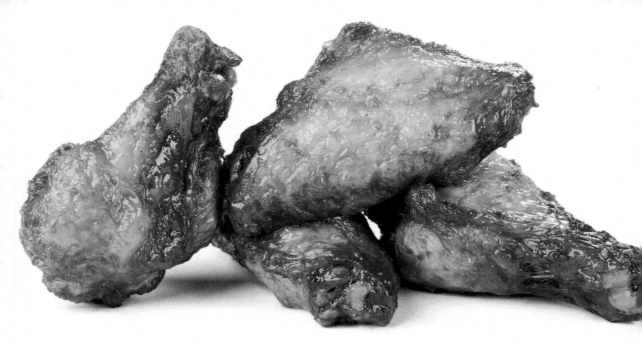

Spicy Chicken Wings

When you remove the wings from the oven, be smart and take your own wings FIRST because otherwise, they may vanish before you get any!

Servings 4

Ingredients

- 40 mixed wings and drumettes
- 4 tbsp extra virgin olive oil
- 2 tsp white pepper
- 2 tsp black pepper
- 1.5 tsp pink Himalayan Salt
- 3 tsp garlic powder
- 2 tsp smoky paprika

Instructions

1. Preheat oven to 425 degrees.
2. Spread all wings on trays with space in between to allow for even cooking and added crispiness.
3. Sprinkle olive oil evenly over all wings.
4. Cover wings with all spices evenly.
5. Bake for 45 minutes. Check after 30 minutes since all ovens have different cooking times.
6. Serve and enjoy!

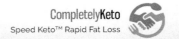

CompletelyKeto
Speed Keto™ Rapid Fat Loss

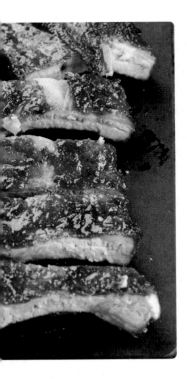

Miami Short Ribs

The name short ribs can be a bit deceiving because beef short ribs are actually quite large. One of these, as you'll see, is plenty for one serving and there is a lot of meat on the bone.

Servings 6

Ingredients

- 6 beef ribs, about 1 ½ inch thick
- ¼ cup wheat free tamari sauce
- ¼ cup approved ketchup
- 1 tsp garlic powder

Instructions

1. Preheat oven to 300 degrees.
2. Grease a baking dish and arrange ribs in 1 layer.
3. Mix all the sauce ingredients well and pour slowly over all the meat. Cover pan with foil.
4. Bake for 2 hours.

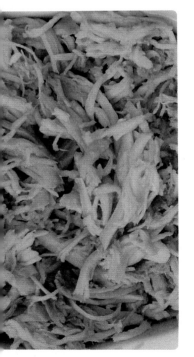

Crockpot Pulled Chicken

In this recipe we use chicken thighs because the meat is more tender than breast meat; however, if you prefer to use chicken breasts, it tastes just as amazing.

Servings 8

Ingredients

- 2 lb boneless chicken thighs
- 1 cup sugar free salsa
- ½ cup wheat free tamari sauce
- 4 tbsp approved ketchup
- 1 cup water

Instructions

1. Put the chicken in the crockpot and pour the salsa, tamari sauce and ketchup over.
2. Cook in crockpot on low for 5 hours, then shred the chicken by pulling with a fork.

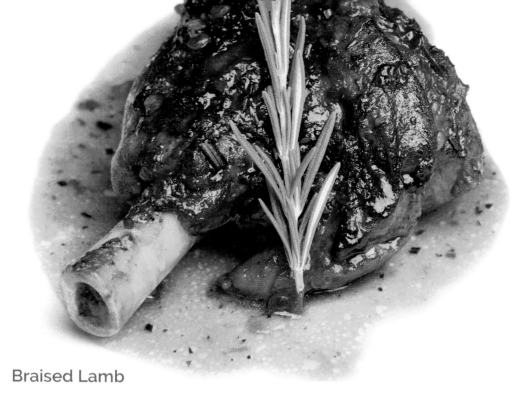

Braised Lamb

Lamb is a delicious red meat that has a taste similar to steak. That's why we are searing and broiling the lamb to give it a nice outer crust.

Servings 3

Ingredients

- 2 lamb shanks (6oz each), frenched
- ¼ tsp dried rosemary
- ¼ tsp dried thyme
- 2 cups beef stock
- 1 small red onion, diced
- 2 garlic cloves, smushed
- 1 tbsp extra virgin olive oil
- ¼ cup Pinot Noir red wine (optional)

Instructions

1. Heat up the oil in a frying pan on medium high flame. Cook the lamb shank for about 2 minutes per side minimum, more if you want less rare.
2. Prepare a baking sheet and broil for 4 minutes, flipping halfway. Remove and set aside to cool.
3. Put the same pan back on medium flame with the onions and garlic and cook for about 5 minutes. Then lower to a simmer and add in all the rest of the ingredients, let cook on low for 45 minutes covered.
4. Pour over the lamb.
5. Serve and enjoy.

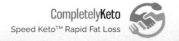

CompletelyKeto
Speed Keto™ Rapid Fat Loss

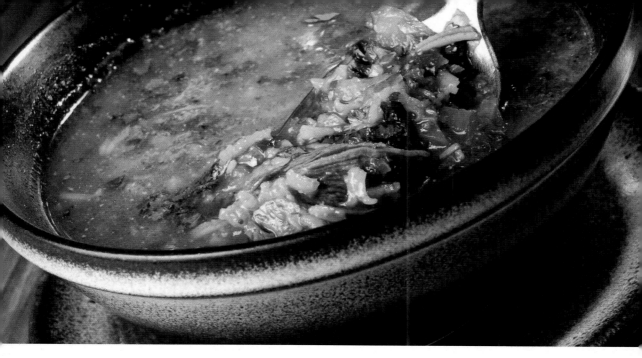

Simple Beef and Vegetable Soup

This recipe calls for water but if you have beef stock available or some sugar free bullion, feel free to add that in for some extra beefy flavor.

Servings 4

Ingredients

- 1 lb sirloin steak
- 1 tbsp extra virgin olive oil
- 1 tsp turmeric
- 1 small red onion, peeled and cut in quarters
- 1/4 small cabbage, shredded
- 1 small zucchini, cut in chunks
- ½ bunch of fresh cilantros, chopped
- 2 tsp pink Himalayan salt

Instructions

1. Heat skillet to medium high heat and add ½ tbsp olive oil.
2. Add steak to the pan and sear 2 minutes per side to form a nice crust. Remove and set aside to rest 10 minutes.
3. Using the same pan, sauté onions in ½ tbsp olive oil and turmeric for 5 minutes, scraping up all the nice bits left from cooking the steak.
4. Add fill water to 2/3 of pot, then vegetables and salt.
5. Cut steak into bite sized pieces and add to the pot.
6. Cook for an hour, then at the end add the fresh cilantro and cook 5 more minutes.
7. Serve and enjoy.

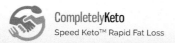

CompletelyKeto
Speed Keto™ Rapid Fat Loss

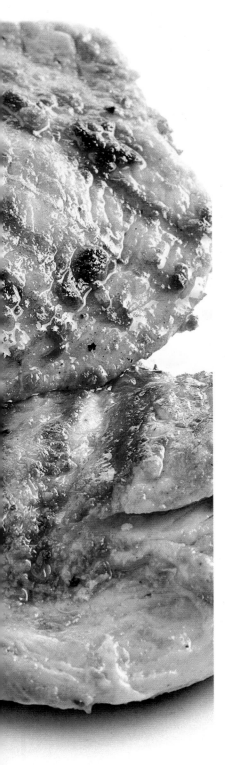

Lemon/Garlic Chicken Breasts

If you choose to freeze these marinaded chicken breasts use a freezer safe bag. Add the marinade and press out all the air then lay the bag and chicken breasts flat on a baking tray. Place the baking tray in the freezer and the chicken will freeze in an easily to thaw package that is also easier to store in the freezer.

Servings 6

Ingredients

- 6 small chicken breasts (about 4 oz each)
- 3 garlic cloves, minced or pushed through a press
- ¼ cup extra virgin olive oil
- Juice from one lemon
- 2 tsp dried (or 1 tbsp fresh) oregano, thyme, tarragon or rosemary

Instructions

1. Place 6 chicken breasts in a large re-sealable plastic bag.
2. Whisk minced garlic, olive oil and lemon juice. Pour over chicken and seal bag. Smoosh the chicken around in the sealed bag until each piece is evenly coated. Freeze or refrigerate until ready to use.

Baking Method:

1. Preheat oven to 350 F. Place thawed breasts in baking dish and bake, on the middle rack of the pre-heated oven for 40 minutes or until the internal temperature of each chicken breast reaches 165 F.

Stove-top Grilling Method:

1. Spray a cast iron grill pan lightly with oil and pre-heat over medium high heat.
2. Grill thawed chicken breasts for approximately 4 minutes per side or until the internal temperature reaches 165 F.

BBQ Method:

1. Pre-heat grill to medium high. Grill thawed chicken breasts until the internal temperature reached 165 F, flipping halfway through.

Crockpot Method:

1. Place frozen chicken in crockpot and cover. Cook for 8 hours on low setting or 6 hours on high.
2. Make sure the internal temperature of each breast reaches 165 F. This makes six portions but... save your left overs for the next recipe!

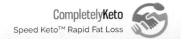

CompletelyKeto
Speed Keto™ Rapid Fat Loss

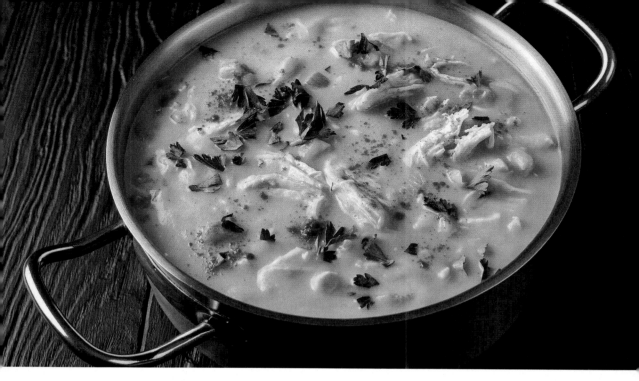

Red Curry Zoodle Soup

In this recipe we are using leftover chicken. We want the zoodles to be aldente, so the steaming hot broth is what cooks the zoodles when poured over them.

Servings 4

Ingredients

- 1 tsp extra virgin olive oil
- ¼ small red onion, diced
- ½ small red bell pepper, thinly sliced
- 3 cloves garlic, minced
- 2 tbsp Thai red curry paste
- 1 tsp ginger, grated
- 1 tsp turmeric group
- 6 cups chicken broth
- 2 cups shredded chicken
- 1 zucchini, spiralized

Instructions

1. Heat oil in a large pot over medium heat. Add onion, garlic and bell pepper and sauté for about 5 minutes until soft.

2. Add red curry paste, ginger and turmeric and stir until combined. Allow the spices to cook for 30 seconds, then add the broth and shredded chicken.

3. Bring to a boil, then simmer uncovered for 35-40 minutes.

4. Ladle into bowls and add zucchini noodles. Top with cilantro and limes.

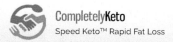

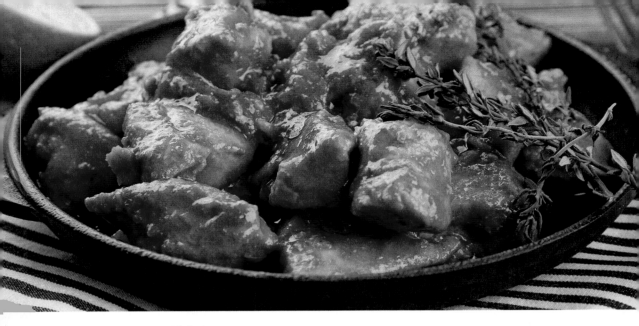

Kung Pao Chicken

This spicy Asian inspired chicken recipe is delicious and filling. The xanthan gum used to marinade the chicken helps to thicken the sauce at the end when the sauce is poured over.

Servings 6

Ingredients

- 1 ½ lb chicken breast, cubed
- 2 tbsp xanthan gum
- 2 tbsp water
- Pinch of black pepper
- 3 tbsp extra virgin olive oil for frying
- 8 sprigs scallions

Sauce:

- 2 tsp wheat free tamari Sauce
- 4 tsp vinegar
- 2 tsp hot sauce
- 4 tsp approved Ketchup

Instructions

1. Put the chicken in a bowl and top with the xanthan gum, 2 tbsp water and pepper. Mix around to fully coat the chicken and let it sit for 2 minutes.

2. Heat the extra virgin oil in a saucepan over medium high flame. Once oil is fully heated, start dropping in the chicken cubes to fry for 4-5 minutes. Let the finished cubes sit on paper towels when done.

3. Remove oil from the pan and add in all the sauce ingredients. Let it cook while mixing until sauce becomes thick, which should take about 3 minutes.

4. Add in the chicken and scallions into the pan then mix around to coat it fully.

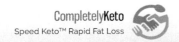
CompletelyKeto
Speed Keto™ Rapid Fat Loss

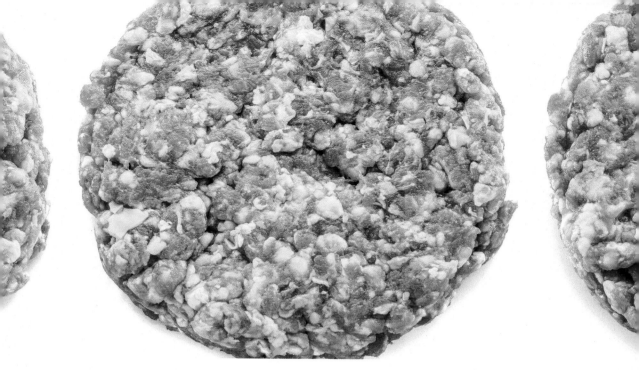

Beef and Cauliflower Burgers

These tasty cauliflower hamburgers are delicious and easy to make. They also freeze well for later use.

Servings 6

Ingredients

- ½ small red onion, diced
- 1 tsp extra virgin olive oil
- 1 ¼ cup cauliflower
- 1 garlic clove, minced
- ½ tsp basil
- ½ tsp garlic powder
- 1 ½ lbs ground beef
- ½ tsp pink Himalayan Salt
- Black pepper

Instructions

1. Heat up the oil in a pan on medium flame.
2. Put the red onion in and sauté for about 6 minutes.
3. Add in the spices and cauliflower then cook for another 10 minutes. Take off the flame and let cool.
4. Mostly mash the cauliflower with a fork and mix with the ground beef. Form 6 patties with your hands.
5. Set oven to broil. Broil for 5 minutes on high then flip and broil for another 5 minutes.

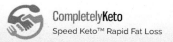

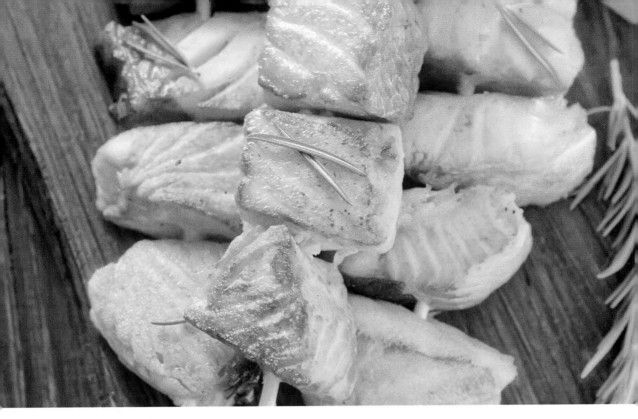

Salmon Skewers

The lime and garlic marinade in this recipe gives the salmon the perfect bright flavor to go with the bite of the crispy peppers.

Servings 4

Ingredients

- 1 lb salmon
- 1 tbsp extra virgin olive oil
- 2 tbsp lime juice
- 1 tsp onion powder
- 2 tsp pink Himalayan Salt
- 1 large bell pepper, cut into squares
- Skewers

Instructions

1. Slice the fish into 1 inch cubes.
2. Mix the onion powder, lime juice and salt in a bowl then coat the fish in it. Let it marinate for 60 minutes.
3. If using wood skewers let them soak for a few minutes.
4. Drain the juice from the fish and thread onto the skewers with the pepper squares in an alternating pattern.
5. Set oven to broil and Broil for 5 minutes per side.

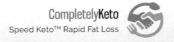

CompletelyKeto

Speed Keto™ Rapid Fat Loss

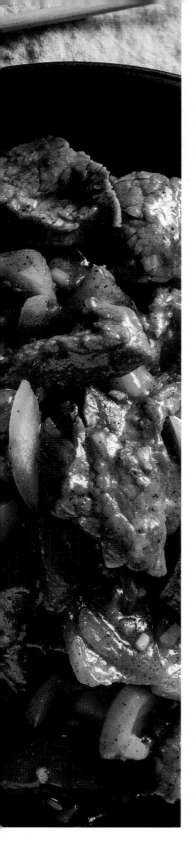

Pepper Steak

This pepper steak recipe is made in the oven instead of a wok. The unique way this dish is cooked gives the steak a much nicer flavor and a beautiful crust on the meat that holds onto the sauce well.

Servings 8

Ingredients

- 2 small green bell peppers, cut into squares
- 1 red onion, sliced
- 2 tbsp extra virgin olive oil
- 2 lbs ribeye steaks (1 inch thick)
- 1 tsp black pepper
- ½ tsp pink Himalayan Salt

Sauce:

- 1 cup beef stock
- 3 tbsp extra virgin olive oil
- 1 tsp black pepper
- 4 tbsp wheat free tamari
- 2 tbsp Pinot Noir wine (optional)
- 1 tsp pink Himalayan Salt
- 4 garlic cloves, minced

Instructions

1. Mix all sauce ingredients together in a bowl and pour ½ of the mixture in a zip lock bag. Save the rest of the sauce in the fridge for later. Place steaks inside and marinade in the fridge 6 hours. Remove and rest at room temperature in the bag for 1 hour.
2. Preheat a cast iron skillet to medium high heat and set oven to 400 degrees.
3. Sear steak in skillet, 2 minutes on one side then flip.
4. Add all vegetables to the same skillet, on the sides and over the top of the steak.
5. Place into the oven and bake about 10 minutes until internal temperature of steak reaches 135°F for medium.
6. Remove from oven and rest 5 minutes.
7. Slice and serve with the veggies and remaining sauce on top.

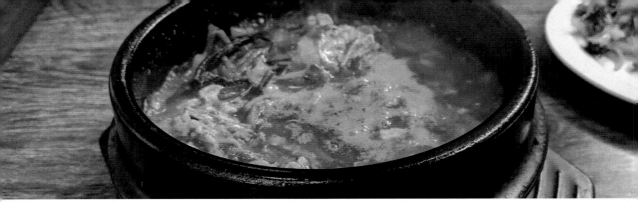

Hunter's Stew

For this recipe I would use a 6 or 8 qt crockpot or slow cooker. Whichever you have would work great to give the flavors time to cook overnight. When it's cooking, the smell coming from your kitchen may make you want to taste it sooner. I like to give it at least 16-24 hours for an absolutely perfect stew.

Servings 12

Ingredients

- 6 strips short ribs, fatty short ribs, bone in
- 6 thighs chicken, boneless
- 6 large eggs in shell
- 2 - 12 oz packages frozen, riced cauliflower in bags
- 1 medium red onion, chopped in thin slivers or cubes
- 2 small or medium zucchini, cut in thick slices
- 2 tsp cumin
- 2 tsp paprika
- 2 tsp cayenne pepper
- 2 tsp garlic powder
- 2 tbsp mustard
- 1 ½ tsp pink Himalayan salt

Instructions

1. Pour cauliflower rice in the slow cooker on the bottom.
2. Add the chopped onions and zucchini
3. Add all spices and mix well.
4. Place eggs whole in shells on the sides of the pot.
5. Place the strips of short ribs on top of the mixture then top with the chicken thighs.
6. Cover with water almost until the top, to give a little space to bubble and not spill over.
7. Turn slow cooker on low and allow to cook between 16-24 hours.
8. When ready to eat remove the eggs from the pot and peel shells off easily. Cut into halves when serving on the side of stew.
9. Enjoy!

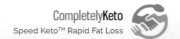

CompletelyKeto
Speed Keto™ Rapid Fat Loss

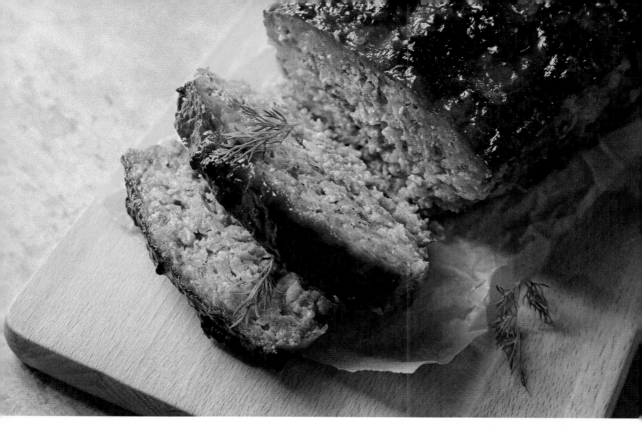

Harlan Kilstein's Meatloaf

This will serve a family. Cut it in half and you'll have 4 meals.

Servings 8

Ingredients

- 10 tbsp approved ketchup
- 2 tbsp apple cider vinegar
- 2 tbsp extra virgin olive oil
- 1 small red onion, finely chopped
- 2 pounds ground beef
- 2 eggs
- 2 tbsp white horseradish, ground
- 2 tbsp kosher salt
- ¼ tsp black pepper, dry
- 1 tsp mustard, dry

Instructions

1. Mix all ingredients together reserving 5 tbsp ketchup.
2. Place in loaf pan. Top with remaining ketchup.
3. Bake at 350 degrees, about 1 hour until internal temperature reaches 155°F
4. Remove and rest 5-8 minutes before slicing and serving

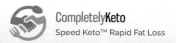

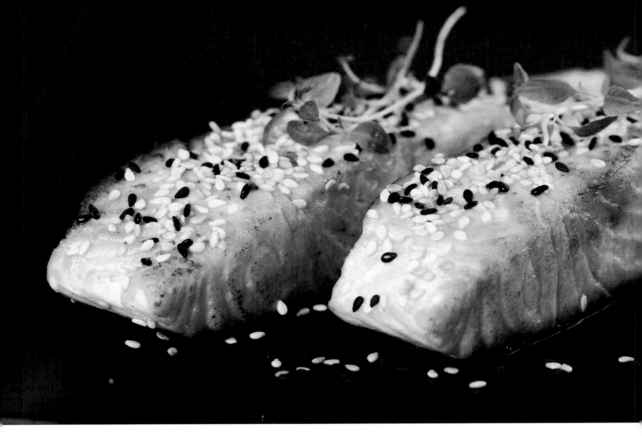

Sesame Crusted Salmon

The sesame seeds coating the salmon in this dish are so deliciously crispy with the fatty fish and bright notes of the mustard.

Servings 2

Ingredients

- 8 oz salmon fillet, 4 oz per serving
- ¼ cup mixed white and black sesame seeds
- Pinch of pink Himalayan salt
- Pinch of black pepper
- 1/8 cup extra virgin olive oil
- ¼ cup wheat free Tamari sauce
- 2 tbsp mustard
- 3 tbsp lime juice

Instructions

1. Heat skillet to medium heat and add olive oil.
2. Mix together remaining ingredients other than sesame seeds and coat the salmon.
3. Then press sesame seeds into the coated salmon on all sides so they stick.
4. Carefully place salmon into pan and cook about 10 minutes turning half way through.
5. Plate and enjoy.

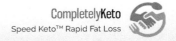

CompletelyKeto
Speed Keto™ Rapid Fat Loss

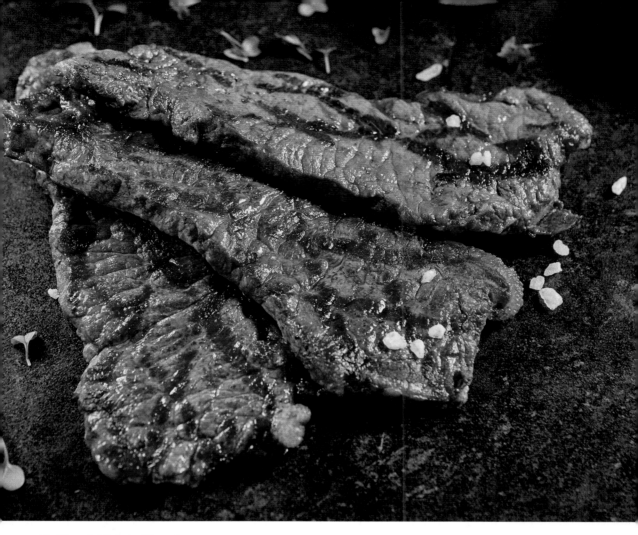

Grilled Skirt Steak

Skirt steak is a bit thinner than other cuts so it will soak up the marinade well and it also cooks quickly.

Servings 2

Ingredients

- ½ lb skirt steak
- Black pepper
- Rosemary
- 2 tbsp extra virgin olive oil
- 6 garlic cloves, crushed

Instructions

1. Place all ingredients in a plastic bag and marinate for a few hours or overnight.
2. Preheat grill to 400°F.
3. Grill for 3 minutes on each side.

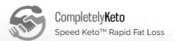

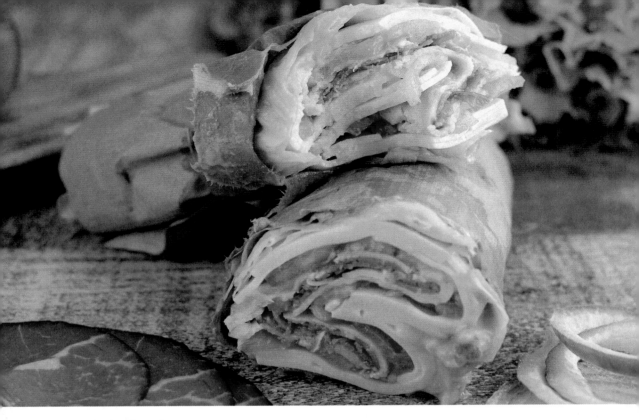

Club For One

This has all the crunchy, savory flavor of a club sandwich with none of the carbs! Pro tip, don't skip the parchment paper, it really makes a difference in keeping your club together.

Servings 1

Ingredients

- 4 large pieces romaine lettuce
- 1 tbsp Primal Kitchen mayonnaise
- 4 oz deli turkey (with no sugar).
- 1 slice red onion
- 2 turkey bacon strips, cooked and cut in half
- ½ small red bell pepper cut into slivers
- Parchment paper for wrapping

Instructions

1. Rinse the romaine and pat dry. Remove the hard stems and ribs and layer the romaine across the parchment paper.
2. Drizzle mayonnaise over the romaine and layer the turkey in the middle.
3. Top with pepper slices, red onion, Turkey bacon.
4. Carefully wrap the sandwich tightly, using the parchment paper to hold it together as you go. Tuck in the sides when you get to the end.
5. Slice the wrap in half through the parchment paper and enjoy.

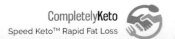

CompletelyKeto
Speed Keto™ Rapid Fat Loss

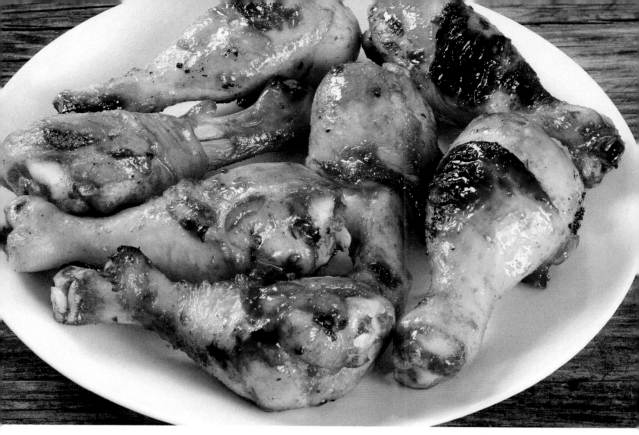

Mustard Lemon Chicken Legs

Mustard is usually thought of as a topping for hot dogs and hamburgers but mustard is often used in grilling and smoking as it gives the meat an amazing flavor when it's cooked in. this recipe uses it in much the same way as a baste while baking. Delicious!

Servings 4

Ingredients

- 4 - 4 oz chicken legs
- 2 tbsp extra virgin olive oil
- 2 tbsp mustard
- 2 tbsp lemon juice
- 2 tsp paprika

Instructions

1. Preheat oven to 400 degrees.
2. Put the chicken pieces skin side up in a dish for the oven.
3. Mix all the other ingredients in a bowl and season to taste.
4. Brush this mix on to each piece of chicken.
5. Bake in the oven for 30 minutes, removing halfway and flipping to coat the other side in sauce.
6. Serve warm for best results.

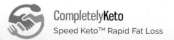

CompletelyKeto
Speed Keto™ Rapid Fat Loss

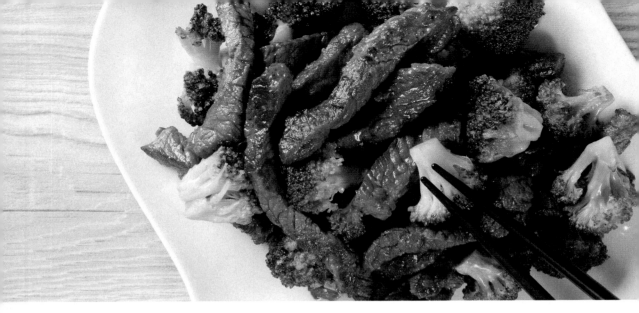

Beef and Broccoli

Since the steak is sliced thin, it will cook quite quickly. Watch the broccoli turn a deeper green. This dish is ready when the broccoli is easily pierced with a fork.

Servings 4

Ingredients

- 1 lb lean beef steak, sliced thin
- 2 tbsp extra virgin olive oil.
- 1 small red onion, chopped into wedges
- Thumb sized ginger piece, minced
- 4 cups broccoli florets
- 1/4 cup tamari sauce, wheat free
- 2 cloves garlic, minced

Instructions

1. In a wok or frying pan add two tablespoons of extra virgin olive oil.
2. Cook over a medium heat. This cooks fast!
3. Cut up one small red onion and add to the pan.
4. Mince 1 small piece of ginger and add to the pan.
5. Mince 2 cloves of garlic and add to the pan. Cook 1 minute then add broccoli to pan. Allow to cook 3-5 minutes.
6. Meanwhile, heat another pan to medium high heat and add beef to the pan.
7. Let brown for a few moments and stir, about 1-2 minutes then add to the pan with the broccoli.
8. Add 1/4 cup wheat free tamari sauce.
9. Continue to cook until broccoli is deep green and easily pierced with a fork.
10. Serve over riced cauliflower if desired. Pour extra sauce over and enjoy.

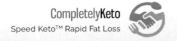

CompletelyKeto
Speed Keto™ Rapid Fat Loss

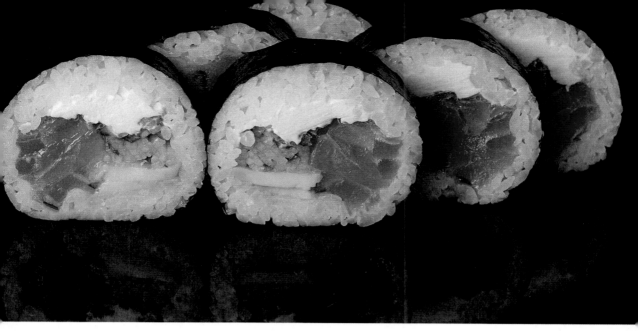

Spicy Tuna Sushi

Thanks to cauliflower rice, sushi is back on the menu! The bamboo roller sheet makes a big difference in easily rolling the sushi tightly.

Servings 1

Ingredients

Spicy Tuna Mix:

- 4 oz Sushi grade fresh tuna, chopped into small bits
- 2 scallions, chopped very thin
- 1/8 tsp black pepper
- ½ tsp cayenne pepper
- 1 tsp wheat free Tamari sauce
- ½ tsp extra virgin oil
- 1 small cucumber, sliced into very thin strips
- ½ cup alfalfa sprouts
- Sheets of Nori Seaweed

Cauliflower Rice:

- 10 oz cauliflower rice
- 1/2 tsp extra virgin olive oil
- 1/2 tsp apple cider vinegar
- 1/8 tbsp pink Himalayan salt

Spicy Mayo Dip:

- 1/4 cup Primal Kitchen mayo
- 1/4 tsp cayenne pepper
- 1 tsp freshly squeezed lime juice

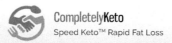

Instructions

- Using a food processor rice the cauliflower into rice sized pieces by turning on and off quickly (check your local supermarket to see the availability of Cauliflower Rice in the freezer section)
- Sauté Cauliflower rice in a pan with the oil, vinegar and salt between 5-10 minutes until water is absorbed.
- Place in refrigerator to cool for 30 minutes
- Put a nori sheet down on a bamboo roller sheet, which should be covered with plastic wrap to prevent sticking
- Spread a very thin layer of cauliflower rice evenly over the entire nori sheet leaving a little less than an inch of space along the top of nori sheet.
- Place Spicy tuna mixture in a row across
- Put a few pieces cucumber strips on top of the tuna mix
- Start to roll sushi tightly using bamboo roller sheet, starting at the bottom end
- Serve with a small dipping bowl on the side using the spicy mayo recipe above

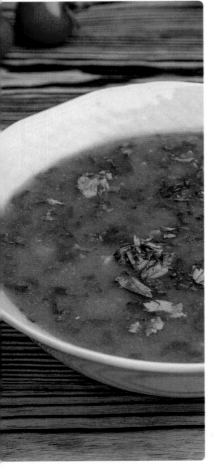

Meat Soup

The marrow bones in this recipe bring lots of flavor to the party. They are packed with nutrients and make the soup taste great.

Servings 8

Ingredients

- 2 green or yellow zucchini
- 2 quarts water
- 2 lbs ribeye steak cut into 1 inch pieces
- 2 small red onions, chopped into ½ inch pieces
- 2 beef marrow bones
- 2 juice of lemon
- Pink Himalayan salt to taste
- Black pepper to taste
- 3 sprigs chopped fresh parsley

Instructions

1. Dice the onions and zucchinis.
2. Put in a large pot with the 2 quarts of water, then add the meat and bones and cook on low for 45 minutes.
3. Add the pepper, lemon juice and salt to taste. Let it continue to simmer for 30 minutes.
4. Remove marrow bones.
5. Serve hot with chopped parsley on top.

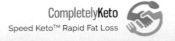
CompletelyKeto
Speed Keto™ Rapid Fat Loss

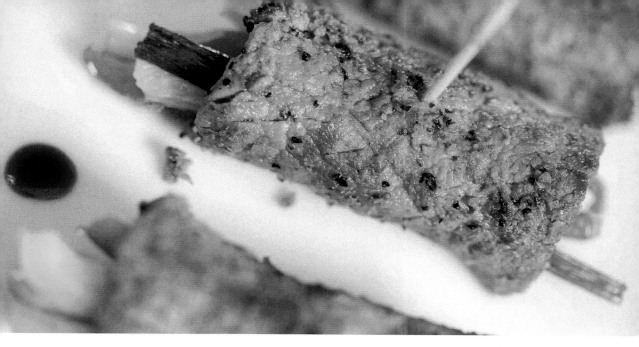

Rolled Steak With Vegetables

If you have a thick cut of steak, slice it to ¼ - ½ inch thick pieces to make it easy to roll around your veggies.

Servings 1

Ingredients

- 4 oz sirloin steak
- ½ large red bell pepper, sliced thin
- 1 small zucchini, sliced thin
- Toothpicks

Marinade:

- 1/3 cup extra virgin olive oil
- 1 tbsp Pinot Noir (optional)
- 2 tbsp lemon juice
- 3 tsp garlic minced
- 1 tsp pink Himalayan Salt
- 1 tsp black pepper

Instructions

1. Mix all the marinade ingredients and coat the steaks in any dish or Ziploc bag.
2. Let marinate for at least 4 hours.
3. Preheat oven to 400 and prepare two baking pans or dishes.
4. Stuff each steak by putting in about 4-6 strips of mixed zucchini and pepper and rolling up tightly. Hold shut with toothpick.
5. Broil on lowest oven rack for 10 minutes.

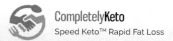

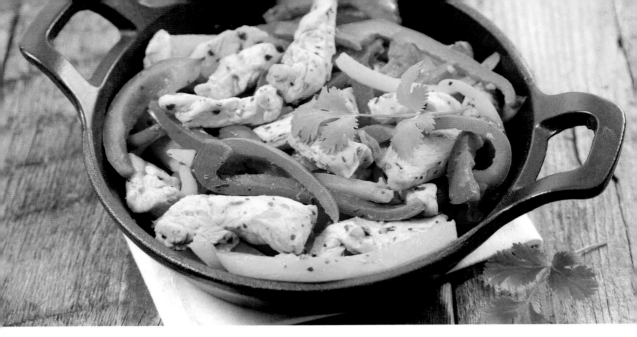

Baked Chicken Fajitas

These are absolutely delicious on their own but also go great in a Crepini egg wrap.

Servings 4

Ingredients

- 1 lb boneless, skinless chicken breasts
- ½ red bell pepper. sliced
- ½ green bell pepper. sliced
- 1 red onion, sliced

Sauce:

- ¼ cup extra virgin olive oil
- 1 tsp garlic powder
- 3 tbsp lime juice
- ½ tsp pink Himalayan Salt
- 1/2 tsp onion powder
- ½ tsp chili powder

Instructions

1. Preheat oven to 400 degrees.
2. Mix together all the sauce ingredients well.
3. Grease a baking pan and lay down the peppers and onions on one side.
4. Pour half the sauce over the veggies.
5. Put chicken on the other side of the pan and pour the rest of the sauce over.
6. Cook for half an hour uncovered in the oven.
7. Feel free to serve in Crepini Cauliflower Wraps

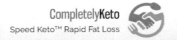
CompletelyKeto
Speed Keto™ Rapid Fat Loss

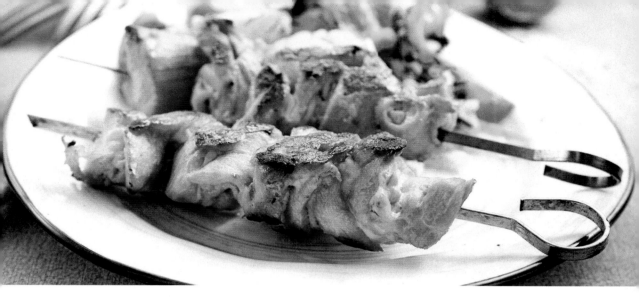

Grilled Herb Tuna Skewers

Tuna is a deliciously flaky and rich fish. Remember that tuna can be cooked like steak. If you like yours just seared on the outside, it's great that way. You can also cook it well done if you like.

Servings 4

Ingredients

- 1 lb tuna steak, cubed
- Pink Himalayan Salt to taste
- Black pepper to taste

Herb Mix:

Ingredients

- 2 fresh oregano sprigs
- 2 fresh rosemary sprigs
- 2 garlic cloves
- ½ tsp onion powder
- 3 tbsp extra virgin olive oil
- ½ tsp pink Himalayan salt
- ½ tsp black pepper
- 2 tbsp apple cider vinegar

Instructions

1. Skewer the tuna onto the wooden sticks and season with salt and pepper.
2. Grill the tuna using a regular grill or a grill pan for about 3 minutes each side, or to however long your preference is.
3. Put all the herb mix ingredients into a food processor and blend.
4. Top the tuna with the herb mix on both sides.
5. Serve and enjoy.

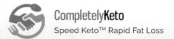

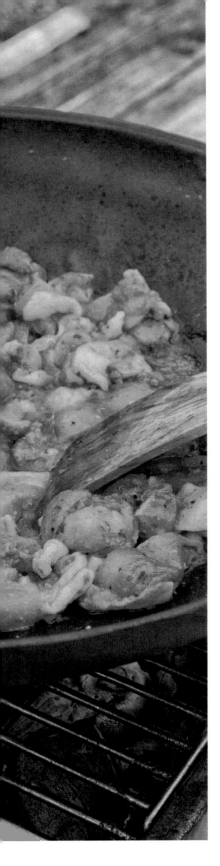

Chicken Pad Thai

This pad Thai recipe has everything we love about the sweet and spicy dish with none of the carbs.

Servings 3

Ingredients

- ½ lb boneless chicken breasts, cut into small thin strips
- 1 whole lime juice, freshly squeezed
- 8 oz Miracle Noodles
- 4 garlic cloves, minced finely
- 3 tbsp extra virgin olive oil
- 7 drops stevia
- 1 cup cabbage, shredded
- ¼ tsp course ground pepper
- 2 ½ tsp pink Himalayan salt
- 4 tbsp wheat free tamari sauce
- 2 large eggs, beaten well
- ¾ cup bean sprouts
- 2 green scallions, chopped in 2 inch strips

Instructions

1. Prepare Miracle noodles according to package instructions and set on the side.
2. Heat a wok or non-stick pan on low heat.
3. Add oil, scallions and minced garlic and saute for 2 minutes.
4. Add shredded cabbage and bean sprouts and stir for 2-3 minutes.
5. Turn heat up to medium.
6. Add pieces of chicken and toss until chicken is cooked through, about 5 minutes.
7. Use a spatula or spoon move everything to one side of the wok or pan.
8. Pour beaten eggs onto the other side of the pan and toss until cooked.
9. Stir everything together until well combined
10. In a small bowl mix together tamari sauce, stevia, salt and pepper.
11. Pour Miracle Noodles into the bowl of sauce and combine well.
12. Turn heat off and add noodle mixture into the wok and stir well.
13. Pour lime juice over the Chicken Pad Thai and serve warm.

CompletelyKeto
Speed Keto™ Rapid Fat Loss

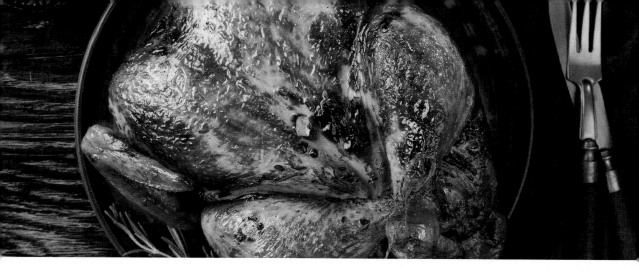

Chicken Filled with Herb Stuffing

The vegetables and herbs cooked inside the chicken are so delicious simmered in the juices and spices. This will be a dinner time favorite.

Servings 8

Ingredients

- 3 lb Whole Chicken

Stuffing:

- 8 celery stalks, chopped very small
- 1 red pepper, chopped into small squares
- 1 yellow pepper, chopped into small squares
- 1 pint mushrooms, cut into small cubes
- 1 bunch parsley, minced finely in a food processor
- 4 tbsp extra virgin olive oil
- 2 tsp pink Himalayan salt
- 1 ½ tbsp cumin
- 1 tbsp garlic powder
- 1 tbsp turmeric powder

Outside chicken rub mix

- ½ tsp cumin
- ½ tsp garlic powder
- ½ tsp turmeric
- ½ tsp pink Himalayan Salt
- 2 tbsp extra virgin olive oil
- 1 clove garlic top, tips cut off
- 1 lime, cut up into wedges
- A few sprigs of any greens to garnish top
- 1 cup water

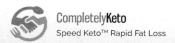

CompletelyKeto
Speed Keto™ Rapid Fat Loss

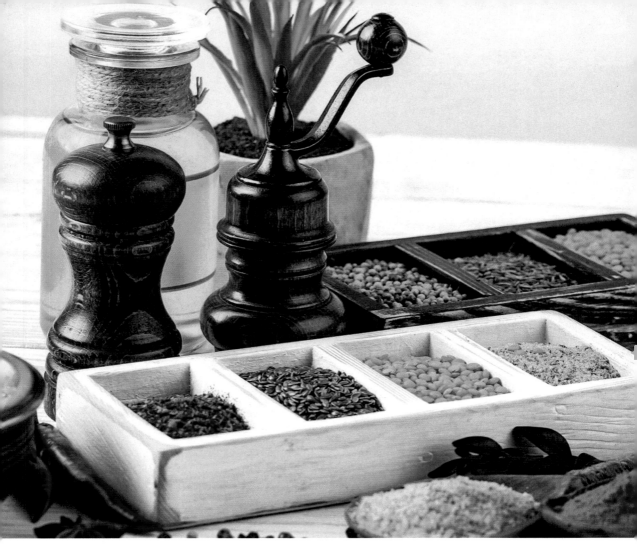

Instructions

1. Preheat oven to 400°F.

2. Place chicken on cutting board.

3. In a large bowl mix all stuffing ingredients until well combined.

4. Spoon all stuffing into the chicken pressing with your fingers to get all of it inside.

5. Place chicken in oven safe roasting pan. If there is extra stuffing spread evenly on the bottom of the pan

6. Mix chicken rub mixture and rub all over outside of chicken.

7. Place whole rinsed garlic head, tips removed, on side of stuffed chicken. Place wedges of lime and greens of choice on top.

8. Pour 1 cup water onto bottom of pan.

9. Roast 1st hour on 400 covered and then lower to 350 for 30 minutes.

10. Remove cover and baste with juices 15 minutes before removing from oven, or until golden.

11. Remove and allow to rest 10 minutes before serving.

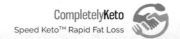

CompletelyKeto
Speed Keto™ Rapid Fat Loss

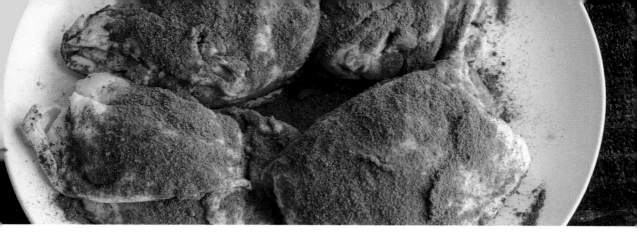

Hungarian Chicken Paprikash

This dish is cooked in the instant pot and the best part is, the instant pot does most of the work for you. There is usually a (meat/stew) option on the settings. If not make sure this dish cooks for 35 minutes at high pressure.

Servings 6

Ingredients

- 2 small red onions, diced
- 3 cloves garlic, minced
- 1 chicken whole 2-3 lbs, cut up into individual pieces (leg, thigh, brest, etc…)
- 1 ½ tsp pink Himalayan salt
- 2 tsp pepper
- 2 tbsp sweet paprika
- 2 tbsp smoky paprika
- ½ lemon, juice only
- 1 tomato
- 1 tbsp tomato paste
- 1 bay leaf
- 3 tbsp extra virgin olive oil
- 2 cups chicken stock or water

Instructions

1. Mix sweet and smoky paprika and sprinkle onto all of your separated chicken pieces. Allow to rest 10-15 minutes.
2. Add olive oil to your Instant pot.
3. Add onion and garlic and turn to saute.
4. Stir frequently for 3 minutes.
5. Add all other ingredients and stir.
6. Lock your instant pot and set it to "meat/stew" then automatic cook. This should cook for 35 minutes.
7. Serve hot.

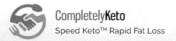

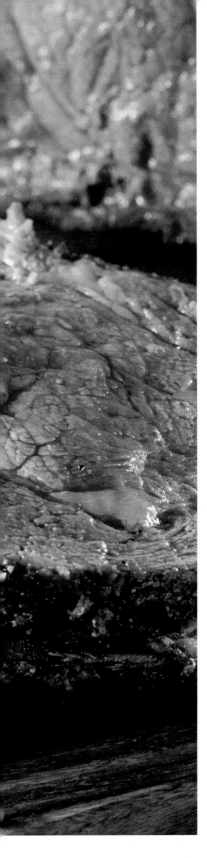

Silvertip Roast (Roast Beef)

This recipe makes an amazing and tender oven baked beef roast to the perfect medium rare. Toward the middle of the roast, the meat will be more rare than the 2 ends. If you like your meat a bit more well done, slice yourself a piece and bake in the oven a few extra minutes.

Servings 16

Ingredients

- 1 large red onion, sliced
- 5 lb Silvertip roast beef
- 5 cloves garlic, crushed
- 1 tsp pink Himalayan salt
- ½ tsp black pepper
- 1 tsp sweet paprika
- 3 tbsp extra virgin olive oil
- 1 tsp cumin
- ½ cup Pinot Noir (optional)
- ½ cup water or 1 cup if you don't use the wine above.
- 1 cup of Harlan Kilstein's Ketchup or Primal Kitchen's

Instructions

1. Place sliced onion on the bottom of a roasting pan.
2. Top with beef roast (rinse off with water first)
3. Preheat the oven to 375°F.
4. Combine garlic, oil, and all spices in a bowl and cover the meat with it evenly.
5. Let it sit for an hour or two to absorb the flavors.
6. Combine the wine, water, and ketchup and pour over the meat.
7. Insert an oven thermometer into the thickest part of the meat.
8. Place in the oven uncovered for 45 minutes.
9. Cover the meat and let it cook until the thermometer shows 135 degrees.
10. The meat will be rare at that time BUT... the meat continues to cook after you take it out of the oven.
11. Let me meat cool for 30-45 before slicing thin.
12. Cover with juices and warm it up in the oven a few additional minutes only if you like well done.
13. Serve and enjoy.

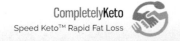

CompletelyKeto
Speed Keto™ Rapid Fat Loss

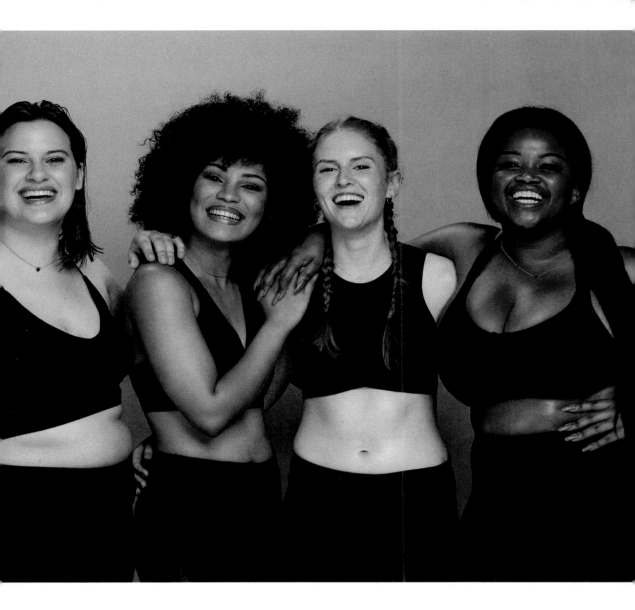

Conclusion

Congratulations!

You've done it. Everyone is noticing the changes in your body. You smile when you look in the mirror. Terrific.

I'm so proud of you for this accomplishment.

When you've achieved success on this program, I'd be so honored if you tell your friends.

If you want to know how to keep your metabolism guessing well into the future, check out my Speed Keto™ program.

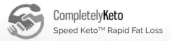

Made in the USA
Monee, IL
18 June 2022

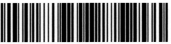

98253938R00055